A Fragile Revolution

Consumers and Psychiatric Survivors Confront the Power of the Mental Health System

A Fragile Revolution

Consumers and Psychiatric Survivors Confront the Power of the Mental Health System

Barbara Everett

Wilfrid Laurier University Press

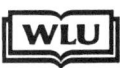

This book has been published with the help of a grant from the Humanities and Social Sciences Federation of Canada, using funds provided by the Social Sciences and Humanities Research Council of Canada. We acknowledge the support of the Canada Council for the Arts for our publishing program. We acknowledge the financial support of the Government of Canada through the Book Publishing Industry Development Program for our publishing activities.

Canadian Cataloguing in Publication Data

Everett, Barbara, 1949-
  A fragile revolution : consumers and psychiatric survivors confront the power of the mental health system

Includes bibliographical references and index.
ISBN 0-88920-342-3

1. Ex-mental patients—Ontario—Political activity. 2. Health care reform—Ontario—Citizen participation. 3. Mental health planning—Ontario—Citizen participation. 4. Mental health policy—Ontario. I. Title.

RA790.7.C3E934 2000   362.2′09713   C99-932342-3

© 2000 Wilfrid Laurier University Press
    Waterloo, Ontario N2L 3C5

Cover art: *Playtime*, a monoprint by Gloria Kagawa, reproduced courtesy of the artist. (View this and other works at http://www.gloriakagawa.com.)

Cover design by Leslie Macredie

Printed in Canada

To my dear son,

Matthew Ferguson

Contents

Acknowledgements

While the production of a book is somewhat of a lonely task, it nonetheless could never be accomplished alone.

Thank you

To my husband, George Roberts, for his obvious pride in my endeavours and his diligent search for typos;

To Judy Varga, who, as the number-one real estate agent in Canada, has no interest whatsoever in the mental health field, but read every word because her best friend wrote it;

To my academic mentors:

Françoise Boudreau for her persistent efforts to make a sociologist out of me. Her love for the integrity of her profession is admirable;

Raymond Morris for his many encouraging phone calls and the lightning speed at which he replied to drafts;

Richard Weisman for his most thoughtful comments and for continuing on despite his bereavement.

To Kathy Boydell, for going ahead and being ever generous with advice and direction when the road seemed uncertain;

To Marilyn Sapsford, who, astoundingly, has become a Baptist minister working in Parkdale. Her reading of earlier drafts provided a touch of the divine;

To Dale Butterill, who diligently soldiered through what she calls my "un-natural" way of thinking, providing insight and challenge;

To the Qualitative Research Group at the Centre for Addiction and Mental Health (chaired by Janet Durbin) for a much-needed forum for discussion and debate throughout the long journey;

To the consumers and psychiatric survivors whose wisdom and passion enliven the following pages:

Patrick Brown	Jennifer Reid
Jennifer Chambers	Marnie Shepherd
Sue Goodwin	Dave Stewart
Paul Reeve	Hugh Tapping
Susan Marshall	Donna
Walter Osoka	M.
Marg Oswin	Mary
Jane Pritchard	John
Paul Reeve	Anonymous

Marilyn Nearing, in memoriam

Introduction

Historically, no one has particularly cared what mental patients have thought about their treatment at the hands of the mental health system. They are outsiders, marginalized and excluded from the social, political, economic and medical discourses that struggle with defining the problem of mental illness and, by extension, what to do about it. Societies are obviously troubled with this complex and seemingly insoluble problem. Over the centuries, they have embraced a number of solutions, each of which started out with optimistic good intentions only to deteriorate into the embodiment of the very difficulties it was supposed to solve.

In the last decade, the Ontario government has been attempting yet another reform of the mental health system. This time, policy makers say it will work because we have learned from our past mistakes (*Putting People First*, 1993). One startling difference between the current period of reform and its predecessors is that government recruited members of a vociferous group of dissatisfied ex-psychiatric patients as part of the early planning process. These ex-patients represent a wider trend, loosely called a "social movement," which is emerging in Canada, the United States and other parts of the world. Some members of this movement call themselves consumers. Others take a stronger stand, calling themselves psychiatric survivors because it is their contention that psychiatric treatment is not just unhelpful but "inhumane, hurtful, degrading and judgmental" (Unzicker, 1989, p. 71).

The first goal of this book is to study self-identified ex-mental patients who, despite their difficulties, lead full and useful lives and who, as part of their activism, lecture at universities, speak at legislative hearings, sit on powerful committees, lobby the government, lead rallies, make films, set legal precedent and on and on—achievements of which most of us only dream. Ex-mental patients, with their new identities as successful social actors rather than marginalized deviants, are a welcome presence in mental health research, a presence that will no doubt challenge prevailing stereotypes. Consumer and psychiatric survivor views on how they have transformed themselves offer fresh insights into the nature of mental health and illness.

Second, the partners of government have traditionally been powerful people whose membership in influential groups and associations ensured at least some balance in power relations. Given the vast power differential between government and consumers and psychiatric survivors, it will be useful to examine what views less powerful people have of the government's initial interest in their perceptions and ideas, and what effect this interest had on the development of their individual and collective identity.

Third, what "crazy" people think has typically been as unimportant to researchers as it has been to clinicians. Thus, an additional goal of this book is to examine consumers' and survivors' own views against the backdrop of the current wave of reform. These new voices offer a fresh perspective on a variety of issues, both old and new. They also challenge and confront a number of firmly held "truths," some of which have been with us for a very long time.

Finally, the theoretical context of the book arises from disciplines known as critical theory and postmodernism, both of which celebrate the utility of multiple voices in the construction of social reality. At the same time, they reject what are known as metanarratives—all-encompassing truths that perpetuate, while at the same time obscure, the mechanisms of oppression (Agger, 1991). Power is central to this theoretical vantage point and, in fact, power relations are just beginning to emerge as acknowledged aids to understanding, first, the workings of the mental health system as a whole and, second, the interactions of its internal actors in particular. The advent of consumer and survivor participation in planning, developing and delivering mental health services heralds a shift in power that is consistent with present-day global trends as identified by Toffler (1980, 1990). In addition, the theorists whose work I have utilized as principal context for the research (Gil, 1996; Janeway, 1980; Wartenberg, 1990) are scholars who are interested in wider constructs, such as political and psychological oppression, new social movements and the path to empowerment and liberation. The application of these ideas to the specific case of consumer and survivor activism promises both to enliven and deepen understanding of this group and its place in the mental health system. It is also hoped that the book will contribute to the field by reinforcing the utility of power analyses in mental health research.

The research questions

The consumer and psychiatric survivor movement will be examined on four levels. Using in-depth interviews with 19 active members from the Ontario movement, conducted in 1994 and 1995, I wanted to understand, first, how ex-mental patients, who bear the burden of intense social stigma, had come to redefine themselves as political activists: consumers and survivors rather than "lunatics" or "psychos." Second, I wanted to know how they translated their personal experiences into political action, both individually and collectively. Third, I asked what they believe in—in other words, what creed or ideology guided their new movement's endeavours. Finally, in light of the movement's increased profile that developed during the study period, the government, at the time, stated that its members were "partners." But how did consumers and survivors characterize their relationship with government?

The subtext of these research questions is intimately related to a power analysis, from both the perspective of individual empowerment and from collective social action. However, in the present context of mental health reform, these processes are evolving under the looming shadow of government—a power relationship that can only be characterized as one of the extremes of inequity. The central intention of this work is to add new voices to mental health and illness discourse, voices that are valuable and credible because, as consumers and survivors so often say, they "have been there."

A word about methodology

I selected a qualitative approach because these methods are particularly compatible with the global nature of my research questions, which address large issues and, as a result, defy reduction to quantitative measurement. In addition, the manner in which the questions are posed calls for process *and* content answers. They ask how and why, as well as what. In fact, the selection of qualitative methodology is a political decision, which is consistent with the theoretical backdrop of the work because it acknowledges the power inherent in the research act. Qualitative methods engage respondents and researcher alike in a liberating relationship with the goal of achieving mutual understanding.

Qualitative methods also demand that I define who I am as researcher, and where my interests lie. I describe my own search for answers, which begins within the confines of my own family, proceeds through my professional experiences of a psychiatric hospital and then veers into the past, where I review historical patterns of reform in the mental health system. I then mine the intricacies of policy, as contained in the Graham Report (Graham, 1988) and *Putting People First* (1993), selecting pivotal words that define mental health reform plans. While I admit that the emphasis I have placed on the contextual background for this research is extensive, it is nonetheless indicative of my intention to tell the whole of the research story, from beginning to end, so that as many voices as possible can speak from these pages.

However, the central voice belongs to consumers and psychiatric survivors. I chose all study respondents from among users or former users of mental health services who developed a profile within the Ontario mental health system through their acknowledged political identity. In this specific case, I sought out self-avowed *consumers* and *survivors*, a group of people whom I see as part of, but not equal to, the more general category of *mental patients* or *ex-mental patients*.

All interviews were taped and transcribed, producing approximately 400 pages of textual data for later analysis. The five themes that resulted from the data analysis process are reported in chapters 5 through 9. It should be noted, however, that it is the essence of qualitative data analysis to look for similarities in respondents' answers while considering dissimilarity to be the exception. It is a common criticism to point out that not *everyone* could have said the same thing or held the same opinion. Indeed, this is true. Qualitative research results require only that *enough* respondents say the same or similar things to produce a theme (Lincoln & Guba, 1985). Consequently, an inherent limitation of these methods is that they do not, nor are they intended to, produce universal truths.

Unlike typical research practice, I offered respondents a choice between anonymity or full identification. Fourteen of the 19 respondents asked that I use both their first and last names when reporting their contribution to the research. The purpose of offering them this option relates to two issues. First, the ideas and analyses offered by this group of people have historically been appropriated for professional use with anonymity as the justification. The choice of full recognition also constituted a political act, signally at least an attempt to create a different research relationship. Second, the nature of the study and the types of questions that I asked were not designed to elicit deeply private material, but rather focused on thoughts that were of a more public nature. As it turned out, respondents often told very personal stories in order to make their points and give depth to their ideas, but even in these instances, most chose to be fully identified. One reason for this openness is that, in their role as advocates, most respondents have presented their personal stories to the public repeatedly at meetings, in legislative hearings or even on radio and television. As a consequence, they see their stories as forms of public testimony and as sources of pride that merit full ownership.

There was a concern regarding identification that cropped up from an unanticipated source. The respondents openly named individual agencies, family members, psychiatrists, other mental health professionals, bureaucrats, their peers and others, and regularly stated their forthright opinions, both positive and negative. Some of the places and organizations discussed were simply innocuous references designed to provide orienting information. However, some descriptions are allegations of misconduct and abuse while others are personal and often acerbic views on specific people. While the study's respondents were free to speak their minds as they chose, I, as a researcher, had no such freedom. Consequently, I decided to respect respondents' views of certain events by reporting them fully while, at the same time, protecting the anonymity of third parties through the use of general category references.

Some caveats

There are three inherent limitations within this work that merit remark. First, it is tied to time. While the research took approximately 4 years to complete, this period is brief when compared with the 10 years allotted to mental health reform and certainly brief from an historical perspective. Since its completion, new developments have occurred which render certain findings prophetic. It is also research that is tied to place. It is focused in Ontario and, to some degree, Toronto, although I made a substantial effort to garner respondents' opinions from other locations in the province. Also, this is a work that examines a particular view of the psychiatric system—a view that has been developed by a group of former mental patients who have come together as a result of mutually defined grievances. Their raison d'etre is critique and, while there may be many patients and ex-patients who profess themselves to be entirely satisfied with their psychiatric treatment, they are not typically among the membership of the consumer and psychiatric survivor movement and their views are not addressed in this work. Third, the study is constrained by who I am as a researcher and who my respondents are in their roles as consumers and survivors. Thus, the final product can be said to be a mutually constructed understanding of the topic which is, by definition, unique. These time, location and person constraints contextualize the study's findings in such a way as to seriously contain extrapolation. Nevertheless, consumer and survivor opinions and relations, as described and discussed by these actors, here (in this place) and now (in this time), have a contribution to make, given the social, economic and political climate in which we live.

1

Nothing changes and
no one gets better

In the late nineteenth century, my great-grandfather left Ontario and migrated west to Manitoba. He was enticed by an offer of free land in return for the backbreaking work of clearing it in preparation for farming. It was a good deal. I grew up on his farm which had been passed on, first to his son and then to his grandson, my father. I also attended the same one-room school where my grandfather and father studied as children.

Prairie farmers, so the legend goes, are tough, independent people who take "nothing from nobody." As with any legend, there is some truth to this one. The men and women in my family prided themselves on making it on their own. Asking for help was a shameful weakness. Of course, what this really meant was that we hid our fragilities and covered our pain. There was a shadow in our background, and in typical fashion, its origin was vague and lacking in substance. This much I know. In the late 1940s, something went seriously wrong with my grandfather. Exactly what happened is unclear because the whole business is mixed up with the kinds of things that families don't talk about. Whatever the case, my grandfather, who in his younger years was remembered as a musically talented, charming, but thoroughly eccentric man, became increasingly erratic, angry and, according to one report, violent. When his behaviour could no longer be tolerated, the authorities were called in and they interpreted his actions as the signs of mental illness. In due course, he was sent away to the Brandon Asylum. No one seems to know what happened to him there, but soon after he emerged, he died.

Every research project has a beginning, and my work on consumer and psychiatric survivor activism has its roots in my grandfather's experience. A hallmark of writing a book such as this is the intensely personal nature of the work because, in essence, I am my own research instrument—both a part of the subject I am studying, as well as the process by which it is studied. Beginning with what little I know of my grandfather's story, this chapter will offer a personal context for my work by attempting to answer the questions, Where am I coming from? and What's my place in all this?

Becoming a professional helper

In 1984, I entered a psychiatric hospital, but, unlike my grandfather, I was not admitted as a patient. Instead, I was hired as a staff member, a psychiatric social worker to be precise. My journey from a farm in Manitoba to a psychiatric hospital in Toronto was a circuitous one. When I finished high school in the late 1960s, I followed a rather predictable career path by marrying straightaway and having a child two years later. I was 26 when my marriage failed. Four years afterward, I found myself thoroughly unhappy with the series of jobs I had held and among the 13.9% of Canadian households that defined themselves as single-parent families living below the poverty line (Gunderson & Muszynski, 1990). Up until then, I had been laissez-faire regarding my own welfare, but when I speculated on how life was about to unfold for my 8-year-old son, Matthew, I stiffened my spine and made serious, concrete plans for the future.

I resurrected the long-dormant dream of going back to university and eventually completing graduate school. As is so often the case, once I made a clear decision about what to do, the minor details, like finances and where to live, fell into place. I put together an income based on child support payments, student loans and grants. I found a cheap apartment near the university and a suitable school for my son. And I got a job working nights as a waitress in a bar. Three years later, I had enough credits to apply for graduate school.

The fact that I became a social worker was in large measure an accident. Getting into graduate school proved a difficult task despite the fact that I had the appropriate grade-point average. Working nights and weekends to support myself and my child left me unable to acquire the well-rounded student experience that would have made me a stellar candidate. Anticipating a difficult time finding a graduate program that would accept me, I applied to anything and everything that seemed remotely appropriate. The School of Social Work at the University of Toronto turned out to be the only program that responded to my application and they were sceptical. Before they would rule on the suitability of my candidacy, I was asked in for a special interview so that they could more closely assess my commitment to the profession. Unfortunately, I had only the vaguest of ideas about what a social worker was or what I might be doing if I became one. When I met with the Admissions Officer, our talk went well and I found myself telling her about my dream of attending graduate school and confessing that, in reality, I hadn't really *planned* to become a social worker, but nevertheless I had worked damned hard to get as far as I had and it was my view that if they accepted me, they wouldn't be disappointed. In the end, I was offered a place in the program. Looking back, it is my hope that I was allowed in because it was understood that having had some life experience was an asset for social work, but the alternative reality is that it was an off year for applications and competition was minimal.

What is mental illness?

At the time I graduated from the social work program, finding a job was not especially difficult. Provincial psychiatric hospitals were a known source of entry-level positions, and when I applied for an opening, I was hired. Aside from the insubstantial knowledge I held in the back of my head regarding my grandfather's experience, I knew little about mental illness or mental patients. Taking stock of my situation, I reasoned that in order to make a success of my new career, I needed to find out, first, what mental illness was and, second, what I was expected to do about it.

On the subject of mental illness, there were two distinct points of view. My professional colleagues felt that mental illness was a chemical imbalance in the brain, probably as a result of genetic factors—interesting news given my own family background. It required diagnosis, medication and occasional hospitalization for acute episodes. *The Diagnostic and Statistical Manual*, the bible of psychiatry as it is often called, clearly listed the signs and symptoms of mental illness, but in its own language: flat affect, dysthymia, ego dystonia, anhedonia—a veritable forest of opaque terms. However, real life was not arranged so tidily. It seemed that mental illness, as observed in the patients, was a catch-all term that meant a lot of things. Some patients had organic brain damage due to some sort of traumatic accident or disease. Some were called schizophrenic, but of that group, some had only had a few psychotic episodes in the past while others were psychotic all the time. Many patients had never been psychotic at all. Some had what was more accurately described as ongoing substance abuse problems. Others had been diagnosed with manic-depression, some with depression alone. A few were developmentally delayed. Some were said to have a variety of personality disorders and others—well, it wasn't clear what was wrong with them. Nevertheless, all received similar inpatient treatment which involved medication combined with cooking groups, life skills teaching, psychotherapy for a select few—most patients were deemed unsuitable for "talk-therapy"—and some off-ward activities like art, music or ceramics. Discharge from inpatient status required staff to arrange for housing, outpatient treatment (usually in the form of a day program) and financial assistance. As a social worker, my job was to help provide personal history assessments, which were documents that essentially told the patient's life story, concentrating particularly on the types of problems that were thought to exacerbate illness, such as marital or familial strife. I was also supposed to help arrange discharge plans. These tasks seemed straightforward. So far, so good.

Things got less clear when I talked with the patients, who provided a second and seemingly oppositional view of mental illness. They said that they weren't sure what had gone wrong for them, but a psychiatric diagnosis coupled with admission to the local "loony bin," as they called it, had only added to the burdens they already bore: sadness, anger, loneliness, abuse and poverty. Although I was far from naive, nothing prepared me for the extent and nature of their suffering as revealed by their life stories. Although there was no such thing as a typical history, most had some combination of the following experiences: sexual, physical or emotional abuse in childhood, gang rape, separation from family due to abandonment or apprehension by the Children's Aid, assault or sexual abuse while in foster homes, assault or sexual abuse while in youth correctional centres or other institutions, alcohol or drug abuse, a series of violent relationships in adulthood, interrupted education, sporadic or no work history, repeated admissions to psychiatric facilities, multiple suicide attempts, repeated episodes of slashing, burning or otherwise violating their own bodies, a history of horrendous living conditions in hostels, boarding and rooming houses, periods of living on the streets, physical ailments associated with poor nutrition and injuries from old assaults or suicide attempts. Patients who were immigrants often came from difficult backgrounds prior to leaving their own countries or, as was increasingly the case, were refugees escaping war-torn nations where they had been tortured and their families killed.

While my own life had not been perfect, it was nevertheless obvious that in the face of this extensive list of disastrous life events, I clearly had advantages. However, I knew something about sexual abuse. The second shadow in our family, aside from my grandfather's trouble, was my father's revelation in his later years that, for him, our one-room schoolhouse had been a place of terror. When he was seven, the School Board hired a young male teacher who did "things" to the boys. My father tended to use 7-year-old words when he talked of what the teacher tried to make him do, how he dreamed that he could get a gun and shoot him and how the dream always turned into a nightmare because, in his heart, he knew the teacher was even more powerful than a gun. He said that as an adult he realized that it had been silly to believe that if he shot the teacher, he would simply get up and continue to come after him. He said, "I was just a little guy. I didn't know." There was, however, some underlying truth to my father's nightmare. A teacher, any teacher, was considered a respected pillar of the community. The boys felt, probably quite rightly, that they had nowhere to run and no one to tell—because who would believe such things could happen? Blessedly, the teacher moved on after one year. Perhaps he felt that if he stayed longer someone would eventually tell. But only the boys knew what he had done, or what he would likely do again at his next school. Speaking of these events was extremely difficult for my father, and thus I knew that it was also hard, very hard, for the patients to tell their stories.

Knowing my father's experience helped me hear the patients' stories—whatever their nature—in a different way. For example, "David" had been admitted to our ward because of a combination of violent outbursts, serious substance abuse problems and suicidal threats. In a talk-therapy session, he related one of many incidents from his childhood. His father was a vicious and violent man who terrorized his family. One day, in a drunken rage, he tied his wife to a chair and began pulling out her fingernails with a pair of pliers. David, who was then a small boy, tried to rescue her and was hit over the head with a wine bottle. Bleeding, but not unconscious, he huddled under the kitchen table and listened to his mother's screams as his father continued to torture her.

Hearing these kinds of stories left me with a set of feelings that I had no idea what to do with. I tried to get angry at the cruel, neglectful families that had caused such pain, but even that obvious outlet was complicated. While it was easy to assume that most patients never wanted to see their families again, in reality, nothing could have been further from the truth. The role of family in the patients' lives was a complex one. In some cases, it was unclear whether a family was abusive or simply victims of circumstance themselves: of poverty, hunger, illness and early death, violence in unsafe neighbourhoods, untrustworthy friends, inadequate supports to assist with children and so on. In other instances, it was the patient, not the family, who had become the aggressor, threatening family members or terrorizing them on visits home. In yet other situations, the family chaos was so great that it was impossible to sort out the victims from the victimizers. Even in those families where overt abuse had occurred, there was usually someone—an adult child, a sister, a brother, aunt, uncle, father or mother—who had shown concern and offered support.

However, the reality was that few family members visited at all. For those who came, the ward was a daunting place and the staff could occasionally be downright unwelcoming, disliking interruptions in their routine. As it was my job to deal with the families, I spent a lot of my time with these visitors. I found them to be confused, distressed, worried and hungry for information. Some spoke no English. Others wanted to help but got tangled up in their emotions, making matters worse. A few, quite frankly, were more disturbed than their relative. Some were tense, angry and blaming. Occasionally, there was a huge upset caused by a family visit that had deteriorated into a fight. But all patients wanted someone—anyone—to visit. Many had lost hope because nobody came.

Hearing David's story and the many others like it raised a lot of questions. There was no way I could deny the persistent feeling that if what had happened to him had happened to me, I would have gone stark, staring mad myself. Was this intuitive knowledge the resurrection of some defective gene passed on by my grandfather? Did David also have a gene for mental illness that preordained his breakdown regardless of the abuse he had suffered? Seeing as I was reasonably sure that I did not suffer from mental illness, had the gene missed me? And if it had, why was I so sure that if I had had David's experiences, I would have gone crazy, gene or no gene? What actually had gone wrong for my grandfather? David? The other patients? It seemed that I had been spectacularly naive thinking that answering the question, What is mental illness? was simply a matter of asking a few questions, reading some books and getting on with the task of being a professional helper. How could I help someone if neither of us knew exactly what the problem was? Despite these questions, the practical reality of my job was that I was supposed to do something about it—whatever "it" was.

Help for the patients

The complexity and the severity of the patients' problems were overwhelming and the distress of their families obvious. The staff's views of what was wanted were clear: stabilization on medication, an application to welfare and then discharge to a boarding home with some sort of psychiatric follow-up, if it could be found. When I asked the patients what they wanted, they told me that their problems would be helped if they had someone to talk to. They also wanted the hospital to offer a safe place to weep and to rage about the bad things that had happened to them. Upon discharge, they wanted a home, a job, a family and friends.

These desires were touchingly simple but enormously difficult to obtain. The ward was neither emotionally nor physically safe. A few patients were unpredictably violent, lashing out at staff or other patients in response to either minimal or no discernible provocation. Even one such patient on the ward left us all on constant alert, never knowing when violence would erupt. The ward rules were numerous and rigid. Their thwarting nature occasioned dozens of verbal and sometimes physical fights between staff and patients, and between patients and other patients. Emotionally, the ward was in constant upheaval and, while there was a lot of weeping and raging, it seemed to be more harmful than healing. A friendship between patients that began as warm and supportive could swiftly deteriorate into insults. Rivalries would develop that might dissipate, or turn into violent vendettas. Patients, often women but occasionally men, were the targets of unwanted and often clumsily aggressive attention from obsessed suitors. Theft was common. At the time, smoking was allowed and cigarettes were a valued commodity. Patients who had cigarettes traded them for favours, while those who didn't spent an enormous amount of time begging for them—often getting a punch from a co-patient because of their incessant pestering. Some of the more vulnerable and disturbed women traded sex for cigarettes.

For staff, the working conditions were unremittingly tense. The ward was mainly staffed by nurses who were expected to take decisive action when violence occurred. There was no outlet for the feelings they must have had when required to wrestle a violent patient into restraints one day and, on the next, resume a therapeutic relationship. There was no formal acknowledgement that ongoing exposure to the constant threat of violence, punctuated by actual incidents, mattered to either staff or patients. Additionally, the men employed in the hospital—whatever their professional role—were informally expected to make themselves available to assist in quelling every violent episode, while the women staff (other than nurses) were expected to respond only if they were unlucky enough to be nearby. Newly hired staff remained "new" until they were assaulted and, after that, they became one of "us." In short, the hospital was hardly a place of healing.

The ward chaos spilled over into discharge plans. A patient and I would work together to sort out the details of getting out of the hospital, but many times our plans did not end well. Co-ordinating the numerous services that were involved in a simple discharge was bad enough, entailing a series of referrals to and appointments with housing, welfare, a community doctor for prescriptions, a daytime program or activity and, sometimes, a case manager. External programs would often turn patients down and the process would have to begin again. If one component of the discharge plan fell through, it placed other aspects in jeopardy. A complex discharge multiplied problems logarithmically. At these times, we had to negotiate services such as the Children's Aid, probation officers, the court system, lawyers, the Public Guardian, specialized services for physical problems, Meals on Wheels and on and on. In order to work their way through these complexities, the patients had to have a head for details, good interviewing skills, an ability to rise above disappointment and, last but not least, eternal patience. In the midst of all these demands, patients would become so anxious they would get into fights on the ward, fall apart in interviews or simply miss appointments, preferring to avoid the whole thing.

All of this activity, if successfully negotiated, netted them nothing that even remotely resembled the home, the job and the friends they wanted. Instead they left the hospital to take up residence in some of the most dismal, dirty and downright dangerous housing I had ever seen—boarding homes in the nearby neighbourhood of Parkdale. Also, people were typically referred to day programs, often called day care, which turned out to be a euphemism for a mind-numbing environment where people sat, isolated and alone, day after day, smoking cigarettes and drinking coffee. Finally, social assistance, the bulk of which went directly to the boarding-home operator, left people living on $20 or $30 a month to cover all their other needs. As a single parent and as a student, I was no stranger to a tight budget, but I had never had to make do in such decrepit circumstances and with so little money.

Nothing changes and no one gets better

Our ward team met twice a week in order to make treatment and discharge decisions. It was extremely rare to have a patient attend these meetings, as it seemed to be our job exclusively to decide what was best. The patients' stories, in the form of various assessments including the version for which I was responsible, were usually well known to most of the staff and, although I could see that some were covertly touched or disturbed by the tragedies these stories represented, the team atmosphere dictated that professionalism meant adopting a tough, heard-it-all-before attitude. Nothing, it appeared, could shock or surprise us.

Discussions of what was best for the patients tended to take three routes, but they all seemed to arrive at the same destination: nothing was going to change and no one would get better. The first approach held that the patients were psychotic, so much of what they said was simply the impenetrable machinations of a diseased mind and, as such, shouldn't be believed. Those who weren't psychotic were manipulative, so they were thought to make up things or exaggerate details in order to get attention. The preferred tactic was to treat the psychotic patients vigorously with medication and ignore or quash the manipulative behaviours of the rest. But, to my eyes, the various medications and dosage levels didn't seem to make much difference, and those who weren't psychotic were adept at outsmarting our attempts at behaviour modification, mainly because we could never agree on, let alone carry out, a unified course of action. So, indeed, nothing changed and no one got better.

The second response was that most of the patients' stories were probably true and, in fact, such horrific tales were ubiquitous among patients in provincial institutions, who were known to be more "difficult" than patients in other facilities. Our patients, it was asserted, were the worst in the city and there was no hope of recovery. Treatment consisted of a change of medication, a change of boarding home and discharge, accompanied by the standard admonishment, "You'll be back." And they came back, regularly, because nothing had changed and life hadn't gotten any better.

The third, less common idea was nonetheless occasionally apparent. The patients had probably brought most of these things on themselves because they were lazy, immoral and a drain upon the taxpayers' purse. What they needed was a good talking-to in order to instil a proper attitude and a solid work ethic. These talks were considered to be therapeutic. The problem was that the patients seemed spectacularly ungrateful for the advice they received, so they never changed or got better.

Control battles

Power was an important factor in the workings of the multidisciplinary team and control battles were constant. Given that staff were free to appropriate the patients' stories and interpret them in whatever way we wished, our *ideas* about the stories became the infinitely pliable medium through which we fought among ourselves for control over the definition of the patient's problem and, by extension, the best treatment plan. Obviously, it was a given that all patients' problems were fundamentally psychiatric ones; however, within this one restriction there was a wide variety of nuances as to the determination of a secondary definition. Would this patient benefit most from help from a social worker? If I could convince the team that such was the case, then I was largely in charge of what happened to the person henceforth. If the problem was more fittingly defined as appropriate for nursing, psychology, occupational therapy and so on, then I was relegated to a back seat from a treatment perspective and my views counted for less. Clearly, a sense of professional entrepreneurship had gotten mixed up in the decision about the true nature of the patient's problem and the best course of action to take. In addition, as the real authors of the stories—the patients—were rarely present in team meetings, they could never contradict a staff member's interpretation of their situation and, as a result, the struggles seemed interminable.

In the end, no matter what perspective prevailed, our discussions were tinged with a deep sense of frustration, often directed at the patients who, unaccountably, refused to improve despite the sincere ministrations of the staff. Given the level of pessimism that surrounded the patients' prognoses, it could be assumed that most team members were simply too angry or burnt out to care anymore—and a few were. But most cared deeply about the patients' welfare and their efforts to help them change and get better were heartfelt and ceaseless. In retrospect, I believe that each of us harboured a different and completely personal definition of what was best for our patients. It was true that our beliefs were related in some way to our professional disciplines with, for example, nurses attending to cleanliness, sleep patterns and regular bowel movements; psychiatrists insisting on medication compliance; psychologists administering personality, IQ and aptitude tests; recreational therapists offering cooking lessons and day trips to local sites; occupational therapists teaching life skills which were intended to lead to some sort of employment; and social workers delving into personal and family backgrounds. However, as I got to know the individual team members better, it seemed that the driving force behind each of our perspectives was more closely related to who we were personally rather than professionally—the things that more deeply defined us as *people*: our own upbringing, our relationship with our children, our gender, our race or ethnicity, our politics and our religion. Whatever the case, team discussions about what was best were intense struggles, although almost always negotiated through a thinly veiled civility where nuances in language and voice inflection were the only signs of conflict.

There was an additional factor, particular to the mental health system, which is helpful in understanding why the patients themselves didn't revolt when their views were ignored or misinterpreted by the team. Under the Mental Health Act, our ward psychiatrist could legally hold patients in hospital against their will and, under certain closely defined circumstances, suspend their right to make decisions on their own behalf. The power that these legal avenues imparted seemed to create a sword of Damocles effect, where patients knew that, should they protest their treatment plans or anything else too vigorously, bad things might happen to them. The idea that one of these bad things could be the legal suspension of their rights was rarely, if ever, discussed. I don't believe the patients had much of an idea that they had any rights. "Bad," as they defined it, related to the rules and regulations that governed ward activities. Suspension of off-ward privileges, denial of visitors, missed meals, struggles over pin-money slips, bath and shower times or transfer to another, less-desirable ward were much more immediate concerns than vague ideas about rights. They were also the ones over which the staff held almost absolute power.

This is not to say that the patients didn't have their own set of retaliation strategies which they employed to annoy staff members, or block, at least temporarily, unpopular decisions. For example, some patients exhibited suspiciously voluntary psychoses with fresh episodes of hearing voices breaking out only when unwanted appointments had been scheduled. Other patients were adept at finding out small, somewhat embarrassing details about staff members which they would announce in a loud voice at ward meetings. One woman drove the night nursing staff crazy by repeatedly tapping on the window of the nursing station. When a nurse would look up to see what the noise was about, the patient would catch her eye, smile wickedly and thumb her nose. As the patient had trouble sleeping, she frequently tapped all night long. A few patients were as talented at psychological interpretation as any psychotherapist I'd seen and, when pushed or thwarted, would deliver a thumbnail sketch of the offending staff member's character that was as razor sharp in its accuracy as it was insulting. Psychiatrists were a favourite target for this type of tongue-lashing. In fact, I found that most of the patients were keen observers of the workings of the staff group and, at any given time, knew the exact nature of the tensions among the team members, tensions that we seemed to think remained behind closed doors. In the end, however, while these strategies could provoke and, in the case of those patients who lost control and assaulted, actually harm, they remained individual protests rather than organized revolts. In fact, staff tended to interpret these sorts of behaviours as fresh evidence of mental illness, although to which disease such behaviours could be assigned was not discussed. However, the bottom line was that the staff were indisputably and irrevocably in charge of the patients' fates.

Who's in charge of the staff?

While patients viewed staff as powerful, the staff themselves did not share this perception. To the outside world, staff possessed all the visible signs of power—professional status, respected credentials and secure, well-paying jobs—but inside the hospital, they felt powerless and controlled. From the perspective of the ward staff, administration seemed to make decisions that were arbitrary, unpredictable and distant from our daily realities—much the same complaint the patients had of us. As well, our ability to affect these decisions or to resist them once they were made seemed limited to non-existent. In an atmosphere of impaired communication, the rumour mill functioned full-time, but as a source of reliable information, it fell short of expectation. Thus, in addition to the often-chaotic ward atmosphere, staff existed in a climate of ongoing uncertainty, unsure as to what administration might be up to that could have drastic implications for our working lives. At the time, observable change seemed to be an exceedingly slow process, sometimes taking years to implement. But this slowness only added to the anxiety as we were ever on the alert, listening for the other shoe to drop.

The hospital and its workings were small potatoes relative to the entire health care system of Ontario which is administered by the Ministry of Health. Politicians came and politicians went, and so, for that matter, did bureaucrats, but no mere personnel change eroded the perceived power of the Ministry. While the staff professed themselves to be powerless in the face of the hospital administration, administration, in their turn, professed themselves to be powerless in the face of the Ministry. As a ward social worker, I can't recall ever seeing an actual Ministry person, and this remoteness only added to the mystery. When senior staff attended meetings with bureaucrats, they always said they we going "up" to the Ministry, even though it was actually located across town. In our world, the Ministry equated to the traditional view of God, all-powerful, all-knowing and unpredictably punitive.

Helpless and hopeless

It didn't take long for me to lose the gloss from my shiny new M.S.W. As far as I could see, the patients had been admitted to hospital with a set of almost insurmountable problems which, they claimed, had been made worse by the ward atmosphere, the lasting stigma associated with an admission to the "loony bin" and the harsh realities that awaited them upon discharge. If all of us, staff and patients, had shared some sort of common language, had been able to hear and talk to one another, we might have been able to agree on what was wrong—bad as it was. Working together, we might have had a ghost of a chance of improving things. To do so, we all would have had to take mutual responsibility. The patients would have had to examine sincerely which of their own actions and behaviours needed to change so that they could have, at least, a shot at an improved life. We, as staff, would have had to understand what life was really like for the patients and adjust our ward treatments and discharge plans accordingly. Even then, it was manifestly clear that there were many, many things that none of us could fix. No one could give back a childhood stolen by abuse and neglect. We couldn't ensure that people were safe in the boarding homes. It was beyond our power to make psychiatric medication more effective, and we couldn't save people from the poverty imposed by a life on social assistance. The benefit of hindsight tells me that we could have *tried* to do some of these things and perhaps, with a lot of effort and wisdom, had an effect over the long term.

In the midst of all this, the clearest and saddest reality was that the patients were desperate for help and we wanted desperately to be helpful. But we couldn't hear one another and, even if we had, we seemed doomed to a continual fight over the true nature of the problems we needed to tackle. No agreement on what was wrong meant no agreement on what to do about it. As a result, we couldn't begin to make the huge, daunting but necessary changes that had to occur first in ourselves, and then in the system as a whole.

All this is not to say that we didn't occasionally have what might be loosely called a success. Sometimes just listening to a patient's pain and rage was deemed helpful. A few took well to the medications and did, indeed, become more stable, although that didn't solve their other problems. Others acknowledged that we had at least tried. We hadn't made a lot of difference, but they were grateful for the obvious effort. Some left and never returned despite the dire predictions that they would do so. I have no idea what happened to them, but maybe they went on to better lives. I hope they did. What the patients never seemed to do was to declare this whole thing a useless waste of time and walk out. They, like us, seemed caught in the mutually held delusion that we would accomplish something, sometime.

In conclusion

It must be stressed that these recollections are filtered through a lens that is particular to me and my life experience and, as such, I make no claim on the ultimate truth. However, they provide one of the backdrops against which this work can be judged. I think it is clear that my experiences left me angry at myself and my colleagues for seemingly making, if not explicit, then certainly implicit promises that we were unable to keep. Had my grandfather encountered the same unfulfilled promises in another time and place? It seemed likely that he had. Provincial psychiatric hospitals have long histories, longer even than my family's 100-year-old prairie roots. Therefore, as part of my quest for answers, I made a study of the history of mental illness—insanity—and I focused my investigations on the hospital where I first began my own professional journey.

2

From insanity to mental illness to psychiatric disability

When I walked the grounds of Queen Street Mental Health Centre,[1] I was accompanied by over 145 years of history. The asylum, as it was called long ago, first opened its doors on January 26, 1850, and the original structure had only been demolished and replaced with modern buildings eight years before I arrived. Aided by the hospital's small archival library, I developed an interest in the history of the old buildings and was rewarded by a parallel discourse on the many questions that my present-day experiences had raised. I also searched for evidence that there had been both patient as well as professional opinions on the topic of mental illness.

Insanity

In 1841, Toronto's population was a mere 20,000, yet the city had to deal with the same sorts of social problems as its larger and older European counterparts. Insanity was one of those problems. Over the centuries, madness had been

---

1 Now part of the Centre for Addiction and Mental Health.

23

attributed to a wide variety of causes: lunar disturbances (hence the term "lunacy"), defects in various body parts, overexertion of the passions, brain topography, or failed magnetic forces, a theory developed in the late nineteenth century by Anton Mesmer of hypnosis fame (Doerner, 1981).

However, there was one theory that came to dominate medical practice. It held that disorders in bodily fluids—blood, phlegm, black and yellow bile—coupled with hereditary factors, were the sources of all illnesses (Baird, undated). Insanity was thought to be caused by an excess of fluid that built pressure inside the body. These pressures were behaviourally expressed as an overabundance of uncontrolled emotion. Relief was promised through vivisection, cutting a vein and draining up to 40 ounces of blood at a time, or through a less vigorous form of bleeding induced by applying leeches. Cupping involved heating a small, thick-walled glass jar and sealing it to the patient's skin so that a vacuum formed underneath. As the air in the jar cooled, the skin exploded, creating large, weeping sores. Blistering was the application of caustic substances to create the same type of wound. Laxatives purged the bowels and emetics induced vomiting (Tuke, 1885). Usually, these measures were accompanied by a near-starvation diet, all in the service of depleting bodily fluids to relieve inflamed passions. A strong sense of moral judgement accompanied these medical theories. The belief was that all humans harboured animalistic tendencies which, if not severely suppressed by dutiful parents, resulted in the expression of uncontrolled emotion in adulthood. Thus, in addition to vigorous medical treatment, the insane were "redisciplined" in the most violent manner as society sought to redress the effects of parental neglect (Akernecht, 1968).

These early theories can be recast in today's terms as a nature-nurture debate. Was insanity caused by an inescapable physiological or biological defect of the body, embryonically confined until it expressed itself as a disease? Or was it created in otherwise healthy humans through exposure to a noxious social environment? This either-or tension, biology or environment, is repeated throughout the history of professional discourse on insanity, although it is a mixed-up debate, often with both causalities resting side by side in a single theory without any obvious effort to reconcile their competing influences. It is also the basis for trans-historical themes in treatment modalities which have focused either on curing a disease in the physical body (nature) or on providing a soothing environment and good advice intended to persuade the mind to adopt clearer thinking (nurture) (Pilgrim & Rogers, 1993).

In mid-nineteenth-century Toronto, the harmless insane were allowed to wander the streets while the city jail, condemned as unfit for human habitation, was converted into a madhouse where the more difficult lunatics were incarcerated. Its first medical superintendent, Dr. Rees, was considered an eccentric man at the best of times, but early on he received a serious head wound as a result of an altercation with a patient and was thereafter himself considered insane (Canniff, 1894). Nevertheless, he remained in charge of the converted jail and followed the medical protocol of the day: cupping, blistering, bleeding, starving and beating. In 1845, Daniel Tuke visited Dr. Rees's jail and reported what he saw.

> It was one of the most painful and distressing places I ever visited. There were perhaps, 70 patients, upon whose faces misery, starvation, and suffering were indelibly impressed. . . . The foreheads and necks of the patients were nearly all scarred with the marks of former cuppings, or were bandaged from more recent ones. . . . Everyone looked emaciated and wretched. Strongly built men were shrunk to skeletons . . . every patient had his or her head shaved. . . . I left the place sickened with disgust. (Tuke, as quoted in Price, 1950, p. 33)

Daniel Tuke was the grandson of William Tuke, a Quaker tea merchant who, upon hearing of the death of a female Friend who had been incarcerated in a British madhouse very much like Dr. Rees's, joined with sympathetic others in order to develop an alternative approach which they called moral treatment. Moral treatment, which favoured the nurture side of the debate, was an attempt to create a utopian world away from the violence and pain of ordinary society. Under its tenets, patients were to be housed within the walls of a small country home called an asylum or sanctuary, where order, kindness, beauty, industry, discipline and devotion to God were to exist in consistent harmony. The asylum's superintendent was to be a benign father figure who lived with the inmates, as did the attendants and their families (Scull, 1979). A sense of family—a new and improved family—was considered to be the centre of this restorative community. Patients were also provided with a set of daily chores which, not incidentally, contributed to the running of the asylum. Work was considered absolutely essential because, without activity, the patients' minds were thought to atrophy in much the same way as unused muscles would.

Moral treatment became the founding principle for the new Toronto Lunatic Asylum that opened just five years after Daniel Tuke's visit. However, it was overcrowded from the start, with violent inmates mixed in with the more harmless and vulnerable. In addition, its Board of Governors had trouble finding a kind father figure to serve as superintendent. The first candidate, Dr. John Scott, was fired when the affair of "the mangled remains of George Andrews" was exposed (Hector, 1961, p. 9). Dr. Scott, hopeful of a job with the anatomy department of the University of Toronto Medical School, was found to have been surreptitiously dismembering the bodies of dead patients in order to practise the techniques of dissection. He was later to find work as Toronto's coroner. When his successor, Dr. Joseph Workman, arrived at his new post, he faced an outbreak of cholera. Inspection of the asylum basement revealed that the drains had never been connected to the city sewer system, and for three long years a huge cesspool of excrement had been collecting under the building's floors (Museum of Mental Health Services, 1993).

During Workman's 22-year tenure, he regularly reported to his superiors that the asylum's physical conditions were wholly inadequate, rendering the building cold, damp and smelly. None of the newly invented mechanical systems intended to ventilate, cool or heat the huge asylum worked and, despite repeated pleas for funds to correct obvious problems, no money was forthcoming. Even more problematic, however, were signs that the promises of moral treatment were unfulfilled. Reports in the local paper alleged that some of the male attendants were allowed to roam the women's wards and that sexual assaults had occurred. In addition, it was reported that a pregnant woman, tied in a straitjacket, had given birth all alone and unaided (Raibel, 1994).

In 1854, William Lyon Mackenzie, leader of the failed 1837 Upper Canada rebellion, sent his daughter to the asylum after his return from exile in the United States. In a series of letters to Workman, he took grave exception to her treatment, and described the asylum as a "gloomy, prison-like dungeon" surrounded by unkempt grounds (Raibel, 1994, p. 391). Workman told him to mind his own business. Three years later, while still in the asylum, his daughter died after setting her own clothes on fire.

The reality of confining large numbers of insane people in the huge, underfunded and impossible-to-maintain buildings meant that moral treatment, as an ideology, was replaced by the very real concerns of asylum management, or custodial care as it came to be called (Rothman, 1970). Custodial care meant that the sole "treatment" for inmates was the work it took to keep the asylum going. Patients worked the fields, tended the gardens, cooked the meals, did the laundry and scrubbed the rooms and corridors. The idea was that vigorous physical labour promoted mental health and vitality. Patient views took a different form. In 1911, Mary A., a newly discharged Toronto Asylum patient, wrote a letter demanding that she receive $1,248 dollars in pay, calculated at $3 per week for the 17 years of her incarceration (Reaume, 1994).

Patients complained that the doctors had no idea what really went on when they weren't on the wards. Clara S. left a letter behind on her chart after a two-month stay in 1915:

> Dr. I am screeming to get ahead of the Nurses as they are bound to cut a patient of their diet everytime they dare to report. . . . I will send you in a correct report of what goes on here among the Nurses. As it is not fair to have everything here reported about the patients. But nothing is said about the Nurses. It is a poor rule that wouldn't work both ways. (Reaume, 1994, p. 403)

Other accounts demonstrate that serious physical symptoms were neglected or misinterpreted as delusions. In 1910, Annie E. died of a strangulated hernia, three months after she wrote the following plea:

> If I lay down to sleep I cannot stay in bed I am up and down
> the Hole night. I feel very sorrow to have to explain all this
> to you but I have been like this longe enough and you Doc-
> tors don't pay the slightest atenion to me were you should
> put the exrase on me and see what is wrong. (Reaume,
> 1994, p. 407)

While moral treatment, as envisioned by the Tukes and
their followers, seemed motivated only by good intentions, in
practice it rapidly deteriorated into the kinds of abuses that
had outraged its original champions. Like the infamous mad-
houses before them, asylums, in their turn, became the universal symbol for cruelty and neglect that formed the basis of a
second generation of reforms.

Mental illness

When a well-to-do, Yale-educated young man named
Clifford Beers wrote about his experiences in American asylums
(1908), people began to take notice. Beers was, in some senses,
the first ex-psychiatric patient activist, but he worked alone,
shunning the company of his fellow patients. With the help of
philanthropists, psychiatrists and other professionals, he
founded his own reform effort, which he called the mental
hygiene movement. Proponents of mental hygiene held the perspective that insanity was a preventable brain disease—a "mental illness," in fact. In Canada, Beers helped form the National
Committee for Mental Hygiene with the aid of a number of
Toronto doctors and wealthy citizens (Griffin, 1989). It was a
precursor to the present-day Canadian Mental Health Association. The Committee's goals were to reduce the stigma of mental illness through public education; to see that returning
World War I soldiers received proper treatment and that new
recruits were screened for psychiatric suitability; to monitor
Canada's immigration policies with an eye to preventing the
country from becoming a "dumping ground for defectives and
degenerates" (Griffin, 1989, p. 30); to provide IQ and psychological tests which assessed the mental health of children; and,
finally, to expose conditions in asylums, one of which was the
Brandon Asylum in Manitoba in which my grandfather would be
confined some 30 years later.

Medical sentiment swung away from social explanations of insanity and embraced a variety of physical therapies designed to treat a bodily disease, now called mental illness. In fact, physicians stated that conditions in asylums were so bad that they were willing to try anything.

> Padded rooms were in frequent use, incontinence of urine and feces was rife . . . some [patients] were extremely violent and tube [forced] feeding was frequent. It was rare for members of staff to walk around disturbed wards unaccompanied. (Cunningham Dax, as quoted in Simmons, 1990, p. 220)

Some of the more popular physical therapies included pneumotherapy (treatment involving the lungs and thoracic cavity); vascular therapy (administering caffeine and other substances to improve circulation in the brain); refrigeration therapy (wrapping patients in artificially cooled blankets and dropping their body temperature as low as 74°F); hydrotherapy (immersing people in baths for long periods of time); histamine therapy (administering anti-allergy drugs); and hibernation therapy (putting patients into a drugged sleep for up to several weeks). Insulin therapy was particularly widespread in the 1940s and 1950s. Comas were induced through insulin overdose and were thought to help people with schizophrenia (Kalinowsky & Hoch, 1961). Doctors also performed lobotomies, which involved boring holes in patients' sculls, inserting a long sharp tool and swishing it from side to side in order to disconnect the frontal lobes from the rest of the brain (Simmons, 1990). The inventor of this procedure received the Nobel prize (Deniker, in Ayd & Blackwell, 1970).

Electroshock therapy, still in use today, was thought to work because of the seizures it produced. Its popularity spread phenomenally and, despite broken bones and some deaths that occurred due to the violence of the electrically induced seizures, patients were shocked as young as 3 and as old as 80 or 90 years of age (Kalinowsky & Hoch, 1961). In the 1950s, a Montreal psychiatrist, Ewen Cameron, developed a theory whereby he postulated that the cure for mental illness lay in destroying the "pathological behaviour patterns held in the memory storage systems" (Cameron, as quoted in Collins, 1988, p. 132). The American CIA funded some of his work because it was expected to provide insight into brainwashing techniques. Cameron combined sleep therapy with intense and repetitive shocks, applied daily for at least a month and often longer (Collins, 1988). The result of such treatment, as experienced by one of Dr. Cameron's patients, was reported many years later in a magazine article:

> [The treatment] put her into a coma for 86 days. . . . When she awoke, the young mother of five had been reduced to a helpless drooling infant. She had no idea who she was. She had forgotten how to walk, how to dress, how to use the toilet. She did not recognize her husband, her parents or her children. ("They Erased My Memory," 1991, p. 102)

At the time Dr. Cameron's experiments were being conducted, patients' views regarding life in a mental hospital were not considered relevant. However, it was fashionable to invite esteemed members of the scientific community, regardless of discipline, to give general advice on patient care, and it was through one of these sorts of visits that a unique insight into the lives of some patients was obtained. Frederick Banting, who received the Nobel prize for the discovery of insulin, offered this assessment.

> I entered these hospitals assuming the attitude that I was one of the patients. . . . I found that the attitude of the doctors and nurses to the patients was all wrong. They treated the patients as inferiors . . . telling them what to do rather than leading them to self help, self-respect, and independence. On the other hand, when the patients were by themselves with a minimum of doctor or nurse supervision, they spoke to each other as equals and were really doing a magnificent job therapeutically for one another. (Banting, as quoted in Griffin, 1989, p. 82)

Banting concluded that, in order to be helpful, mental hospitals had to radically change their policies and procedures, but the mental hygiene movement was in firm pursuit of a medical solution to the problem of mental illness and his advice was not taken.

In the end, Clifford Beers lost momentum. He became preoccupied with trying to prove to his upper-class followers that he was, indeed, sane (Dain, 1980). In the latter years of his life he spent time in private asylums, and he passed away before the effects of his movement could be fully assessed. In fact, the mental hygiene movement's involvement in the treatment of returning troops and the screening of soldiers in both world wars helped legitimize the value of psychiatric treatment and expand psychiatry's role beyond the boundaries of the asylum (Grob, 1991). In Ontario, movement members secured funding for the establishment of psychiatric wards in general hospitals and a network of outpatient clinics (Blom & Sussman, 1989). Employment opportunities for psychiatrists and other mental health professionals grew exponentially. Also, members conducted a number of studies on Japanese Canadians and Ukrainian Canadians in search of "the immigrant with a lame or crippled mind" (Reid, as quoted in Griffin, 1989, p. 96), an activity that tied some mental hygiene ideas directly to those of the now-reviled eugenics movement. However, while it might be argued that the movement offered people a new and, some would say, more respectful language with which to discuss the insane (the mentally ill), the reality was that the public's attitudes remained as negative as ever. Further, the movement's focus on the early detection and treatment of mental illness as a prevention measure had the unintended effect of promoting psychiatric hospitalization among the middle classes, who had heretofore largely escaped the psychiatric gaze (Carrol, 1964). And, as a final blow, complaints of abuses within institutions multiplied, indicating that conditions had actually worsened during this particular period of reform (Dain, 1980).

In the welcoming public atmosphere that the mental hygiene movement created for psychiatry, the damaging nature of many of its physical treatments went unnoticed. In fact, continued development of the biological view of mental illness became "inextricably linked to a professional strategy of collective upward mobility" (Pilgrim & Rogers, 1993, p. 105). Eventually, however, these sorts of treatments gave way to new biochemical technologies, allowing big business, in the form of pharmaceutical companies, to enter the mental illness equation for the first time.

With the introduction of psychotropic medications, it was generally felt that psychiatry was at last on the right path. The rise of both the physical and chemical therapies cast the old Toronto Asylum in a new light. It was no longer considered a custodial care facility where crazy people were kept indefinitely, but a modern hospital for the treatment of mental illness. In honour of its new role, it was renamed for its address: 999 Queen Street West or, as it became known locally, simply 999.

Anti-psychiatric thought and feminist criticism

The new emphasis on psychiatry and the biochemistry of mental illness was offset by a developing field of alternative thought called anti-psychiatry, a collection of views that favoured the nurture side of the mental illness debate and tended to advocate for the talk therapies (psychotherapy and psychoanalysis, for example) rather than drugs and shock treatment.

It can be argued that Freud opened the door to criticism. His own theories of psychoanalysis eventually found a welcoming home within psychiatric discourse once he dropped the idea that his women patients had *actually* experienced incest and began publicly to relabel their stories as fantasies (Herman, 1992). With Freud came the idea that the unconscious, the unseeable mind, could make you mentally ill, and talk, which revealed the hidden pathology, could make you well. At the same time, the plight of returning veterans from both world wars discredited psychiatry's central idea: all mental illness was the product of genetic factors. The trauma of battle had clearly produced the classic symptoms of "disease" in heretofore healthy young men from fine families and, as a consequence, the role of environmental factors in the etiology of mental distress took on heightened meaning (Pilgrim & Rogers, 1993).

The first widely recognized challenge to psychiatry came from R.D. Laing, who, in *The Divided Self* (1960), published persuasively written case studies of his women patients. His basic thesis was that the delusions associated with schizophrenia were not produced by illness, but instead had a perfectly intelligible explanation which could be found in the abuse the patient had suffered at the hands of his or her family. Laing's associate, David Cooper, was the first to call these new ideas "anti-psychiatry" because he argued that the coercive and hypocritical aspects of family life were simply reproduced in the power and trickery exercised by psychiatrists. Laing, an abused child himself, defined schizophrenia as a misunderstood but noble state of being characterized by insight or even prophecy. He argued that people with schizophrenia did not require institutionalization, drugs or shock treatment. Instead, they needed respect and nurturance until their psycho-spiritual crises passed.

In the 1960s, Laing and his colleagues established Kingsley Hall, located in East London. Here, they endeavoured to put their ideas into practice. Kingsley Hall encouraged visits from rock stars, actors and other celebrities, but its ability to heal its patients was limited in the chaos of what appeared to be an ongoing party, highlighted by a regular late-night event called the lunatics' ball. In the 1970s, burnt out from alcohol and drug abuse, Laing recanted his earlier theories, denying that he had ever thought of himself as anti-psychiatry and even offering a kind word for electric shock treatment. David Cooper further disgraced the group by advocating for what he called "bed therapy." In published papers, he openly admitted to having sex with his women patients, justified as an attempt to deepen his spiritual connection with them (Showalter, 1985).

However, the anti-psychiatry perspective had other sources of life. In 1961, Goffman published his analysis of life in what he called a "total" institution. In his famous book *Asylums*, he stepped metaphorically into the shoes of a mental patient, taking readers through a psychiatric hospital experience as seen through his male, white, middle-class eyes. Goffman was a skilled writer and readers were drawn into the life of his fictional patient so that they, too, felt his dawning horror when, abandoned by his family in what at first appears to be a benign and caring hospital, he is inexorably enveloped in the degradation and humiliation of psychiatric treatment. Readers struggle along with the patient to preserve dignity and identity. And, when the patient is defeated, they feel his pain and his loss.

Thomas Scheff (1966) added his voice to the rising tide of criticism by proposing that mental illness existed chiefly in the eye of the beholder. His studies sought to support labelling theory, a body of thought which held that psychiatric symptoms were not a manifestation of disease, but instead were contextual, appearing and disappearing according to the social milieu in which patients found themselves. Patients' labels—their diagnoses—were a shorthand language developed by psychiatrists to identify people who behave differently from the dominant classes. Labels also justified remedial action so that these behaviours could be suppressed through incarceration and so-called treatment. Labelling theorists wanted to demonstrate that it was principally the luck of the draw that dictated whether deviant persons came to be called mad or bad.

Thomas Szasz (1974) attacked psychiatric practice as an infringement on individual civil liberties. He defined the legal powers of psychiatry as "the armed hunt for happiness of the Other" and, as such, the most dangerous of delusions (Szasz, 1989, p. xv). According to him, mental illness does not exist. Instead, it is an elaborate metaphor to justify psychiatry's real role, which is to rid society of an extremely difficult class of people. Psychiatry's deception can be seen in the paradox of its powers. On one hand, the profession imprisons supposedly mentally ill persons when there is no evidence of criminal activity, while, on the other, it colludes with the state by finding them not guilty when it is clear that they have committed a crime. Szasz contends that if psychiatry were stripped of its powers to suspend its patients' civil rights and to participate in the insanity defense, it would simply cease to exist.

The rise of feminism added another perspective to the psychiatry versus anti-psychiatry debate. Women scholars were suspicious of the male-as-all-powerful-therapist theme that ran through anti-psychiatry thinking, and they deplored the fact that some proponents openly exploited women patients with impunity. Thus, feminists developed their own distinct analyses that attacked psychiatry through the lens of gender. Chesler (1972) charged that psychiatry had been instrumental in silencing women who did not conform to the standard social roles that had been assigned to them. Using Elizabeth Packard as an example (a woman confined in an asylum in 1860 by her clergyman husband for expressing religious opinions that disagreed with his), Chesler developed the idea that asylums were used as punishment for rebellious women. She charged that the abuses they suffered while incarcerated were simply extensions of those experienced by most women in a patriarchal society. Penfold and Walker (1983) dissected psychiatry from inside the profession. They argued that, because there is no diagnostic test or observable lesion associated with mental illness, diagnoses are merely opinions, but opinions that carry enormous weight. To be *called* crazy by a so-called expert is to *be* crazy. In short, the language of psychiatry manufactures its own reality which can encircle women, allowing them no exit from the dilemma it has itself created.

While anti-psychiatry theorists, feminists and others are highly critical of the psychiatric paradigm and the physical treatments it spawns, the talk therapies for which they so strongly advocate are not themselves exclusively benign or non-invasive. Certainly, one very serious problem is the potential for sexual and emotional exploitation. A second concern is the bane of any treatment modality: the talk therapy practitioner may be incompetent, unskilled or employing a flawed theoretical framework (Pilgrim & Rogers, 1993). Indeed, from the perspective of the actual patient, psychiatry and anti-psychiatry treatments may not be as far apart as they appear to the protagonists. Each identifies the patient or client as a victim, either of disease or environment. In both instances, rescue is achieved only through professional intervention and, finally, each form of treatment can be offered with dedication and kindness or with cruelty and abuse.

The therapeutic community

These sorts of vigorous debates created a climate of optimism and excitement at 999 Queen Street West where, in the early 1970s, staff embraced a short-lived treatment movement—at least in the field of psychiatry—called the therapeutic community. It was an idea that reworked moral treatment's emphasis on the social causes of mental illness and was championed by Maxwell Jones, a British psychiatrist who was employed in the treatment of World War II soldiers who had broken down in combat. He developed the idea of a therapeutic community which, like moral treatment, sought to provide a restorative environment where patients (he prophetically called them consumers) would learn socially more acceptable behaviours so that they could fit into life outside the hospital.

Maxwell Jones spent many months in Toronto, influencing administration and teaching the new way (Dukszta, 1987). In a therapeutic community, patients were reconceptualized as active agents in their own treatment and accorded the right to question the ideas and decisions of professional staff (Jones, 1973). The hospital environment was supposed to resemble the real world as much as possible so that patients would be able to use their learning upon discharge.

While I was still working at the hospital, I took the opportunity of interviewing some of the longer-term patients, asking what they thought about the days of the therapeutic community. "Rosie," a frequent inpatient during this time, describes her experience this way:

> When you came in, you were assigned to a group. One of the patients who was together—not someone who had just gotten admitted and who was out to lunch—would introduce themselves to you and you to them. Now, right away you feel better. You're not surrounded by staff because the paranoia really hits you when that happens. Then they would take you and orient you. This is the cafeteria. This is your room, and so on. And they were your buddy. The patients manned the front desk, taking turns for a couple of hours a day and we never lost a patient. We knew who had privileges and who didn't. (*Rosie*, 1988)

Rosie also reported that one of the skills she learned as a result of the therapeutic community was the ability to negotiate quid pro quo agreements among the patients on front-desk duty. For example, she would be allowed to slip out in the evenings and spend an hour or two in the bar across the street without the staff ever knowing if, when it was her turn for duty, she would extend the same courtesy to her fellows. Thus, the therapeutic community was teaching Rosie a set of skills, probably other than what was intended, but nevertheless she judged it to be a helpful and benign environment. In fact, after a 20-year association with the hospital, Rosie considered the therapeutic community to be the "good old days" of inpatient treatment.

However, on the international stage, criticisms of the therapeutic community were heating up, charging mainly that the skills inpatients learned had no particular validity in the real world (Pilgrim & Rogers, 1993). In the early 1980s, a set of tragic events suddenly intervened at 999 Queen Street when three patients died due to accidental staff-administered overdoses of medication. Soon, a team of consultants was commissioned to look into conditions (Simmons, 1990). The resulting operational review blamed the therapeutic community. The consultants felt that the model, which discouraged locked wards and mechanical restraints, underemphasized security. Among other things, the report recommended a more scientific approach to patient care, the centralization of administration and management functions, the reinstitution of mechanical restraint and the creation of locked wards (Peat, Marwick & Partners, 1982).

Deinstitutionalization

In concert with this damning report was the emerging notion that institutions caused more problems than they solved—the exact inverse of the thinking that had created asylums in the first place. The new philosophy, called deinstitutionalization, was summed up by Cohen (1985) as, "small is beautiful, people are not machines, experts don't know everything, bureaucracies are anti-human, institutions are unnatural and bad, the community is natural and good" (p. 35).

In the case of the 125-year-old building that was the original Toronto Lunatic Asylum, deinstitutionalization was a literal as well as philosophical threat. The huge structure was showing serious signs of age and, while local historical preservation foundations fought valiantly to save it, it was scheduled for demolition. Even with its new status as a modern hospital and its new name, 999 Queen Street West, the old building's public image was one of fear and ridicule: 999 was the funny farm, the loony bin. A local columnist wrote at the time:

> So they want to save 999. They can't have ever been there.
> For if you were there once, you would not need to preserve
> the building. You would never forget it. I can sit here now,
> surrounded by light and warmth and companionship and
> recreate that monstrous building, even though it was years
> since I was there. There are the sounds. The heavy clang of
> doors shutting some in and some out: the rattle of the keys
> that in turning brought the outside world in and then
> closed it off. Those were the sounds of 999. I will never for-
> get them. There were the sights: barbaric reminders of
> human indignity, human indifference, callousness. But
> mostly 999 was a smell. If you were never there, I hope you
> never smell that smell. But if you were, it will never leave
> your nostrils. Saving 999. Why? I wonder. (Sutton, *Toronto
> Sun*, December 17, 1975, as quoted in Baird, undated)

Efforts to interest the government in preserving the old
asylum as an architectural artefact failed, and the wrecker's
ball brought it down. New, smaller, modern buildings were
erected on the site and the hospital was, once again, renamed
and its address changed in search of a new image. It became
Queen Street Mental Health Centre, located at 1001 Queen
Street West.

It is often said that the true basis for this movement was
the discovery of psychiatric medication, but the reality was that
institutions began to close before medications became readily
available (Pilgrim & Rogers, 1993; Simmons, 1990). The budgets
of the remaining institutions consumed as much as the whole
system had before (Minkhoff, 1987), partially because of a 300%
increase in the number of professionals they employed (Lurie,
1984). In fact, many of the patients weren't deinstitutionalized
at all, but instead were simply transferred to nursing homes or
other provincially funded residential facilities (Lurie, 1984).
Also, for those who were discharged, the "good" community
wasn't as welcoming as had been hoped. Many of the newly
released patients, facing life in filthy and run-down boarding
homes, deteriorated further. Attempts to return them to the
institution, coupled with decreasing lengths of stay, created
what was called the revolving door syndrome (Minkhoff, 1987).
Other ex-patients simply took their chances on the streets.

Psychiatric disability

The last professional discourse to be discussed in this chapter is a contemporary one, and as such remains a work in progress. In the United States, as a response to deinstitutionalization, the Kennedy administration formally created what was supposed to be a network of community mental health services located outside of hospitals.

The idea that mental patients require "rehabilitation" for their "psychiatric disability" grew out of Boston University in the early 1970s, championed by William Anthony. Just like people who have suffered a severe physical injury and find themselves confined to a wheelchair, for example, people with psychiatric disabilities are thought to need new skills so that they can live, work and learn in the environment of their choice (Anthony, Cohen & Farkas, 1990). Also, communities themselves are supposed to change so that the psychiatrically disabled can be accommodated. Accommodation, in this case, is defined as convincing employers to give the mentally ill a chance, lobbying for funding for subsidized housing and community mental health programs and attempting to involve or reinvolve family and friends in the disabled person's life.

In Ontario, the use of the term psychiatric rehabilitation or, as it is sometimes called, psychosocial rehabilitation, is less pervasive. Instead, being ever practical, we Canadians tend to call community mental health services just what they are— community mental health services. These programs, which are typically composed of non-medical services such as supportive housing, case management, drop-in centres, workshops and crisis services, have developed willy-nilly over the past three decades in accordance with the abilities of individuals or communities to promote their ideas to government funders (Boydell, 1996).

Community mental health services are a relatively new development when viewed in the context of this historical review. Nevertheless, a critique has arisen. John McKnight (1994), a long-time American community organizer and activist, argues that social services, including the mental health variety, appropriate people's ability to define their own problems and to develop their own solutions. He believes that, just like traditional psychiatry, community services simply find more and more problems to justify their proliferation, or, as Cohen (1985) says, "cast wider, stronger and different nets" (p. 38).

In conclusion

Unlike the reforms that populate the history of mental health, the present period of change in Ontario has arisen at a time when ex-mental patients have for the first time entered the picture in substantial numbers. While their forebears tended to confine themselves to pleading for better and fairer treatment at the hands of their keepers, this new breed of activist seems to be taking a different approach. They are often well versed in the history of psychiatry and almost always knowledgeable about current professional discourse. Through the telling and retelling of their own experiences of mental health treatment, they are intent upon making their voices heard. Their very presence in this period of mental health reform heralds a shift in power. In fact, they contend that power and its uses are what is at the bottom of it all (Burstow, 1992).

3

Power and protest

Many years after the completion of his famous text *Madness and Civilization* (1965), Foucault decided that the history of psychiatry is, in fact, a genealogy of power, but he expresses regret that he failed to recognize it at the time (1977). My own experience as a staff member in a contemporary psychiatric hospital bears personal witness to an ongoing struggle among a set of power relationships in which the patients, staff, administrators and the Ministry were embedded. It appeared that everyone felt powerless in relation to some more powerful entity and, while the patients clearly needed help and the staff wanted to be helpful, not much seemed to work.

Foucault (1994a) argues that it is not enough to identify the existence of a struggle and just leave it at that. Instead, it is necessary to ask what we are struggling over. Who is involved? How, where, by what means and according to what rationale has the struggle evolved? The benefit of hindsight makes it possible to offer some answers to these questions. In the case of mental illness, the people who have historically been most involved in the debate have tended to be society's elite: the well educated, those holding professional status, sometimes philanthropists, often politicians or government officials. These are powerful people, and it is their ideas that have shaped our notion of what mental illness is and what to do about it. The battleground has been the drawing rooms of the

wealthy, the academic classroom, medical journals and government legislatures. What have we been struggling over? Foucault (1994b) states that "we are subjected to the production
of truth through power and we cannot exercise power except
through the production of truth" (p. 31). In our society, the
truth is often purveyed to us through the medium of erudite
knowledge: in this instance, formally produced and sanctioned
theories about how mental illness is caused and how it might
be cured. The stated rationale for the production of these theories has been the desire on the part of the elite strata of society
to be helpful to those who are suffering. However, the critics of
psychiatry argue that, in reality, this form of helping is merely a
thinly disguised justification for locking troublesome people
away so they don't annoy us. Dain (1980) insists that each era of
reform amounted simply to a series of improved methods for
social control, principally because those directing the changes
were from the same social classes and groups as those perpe-
trating (or ignoring) the abuses. In fact, the medical and psychiatric enterprise has often been likened to a self-sustaining
industry that, at one and the same time, produces a diagnosis
of illness, and then offers to treat or cure it (Albrecht, 1992;
Gadacz, 1994).

Whatever the ascribed motivation, the erudite discourse
that has evolved around mental illness has been an ebb and flow
of explanations that alternately emphasize physical disease or
social causalities—nature versus nurture. Anti-psychiatry proponents and feminists have recast the debate in contemporary
terms and have added a dimension to our understanding, but
the alternative treatments they propose have also demonstrated a potential for abuse and exploitation. The debate has
proven itself to be repetitive and circular because it is the same
classes of people continually arguing point and counterpoint.

While the rhetoric of how to cure or ameliorate insanity,
mental illness or psychiatric disability has been a hotly contested area of struggle, a conspicuously missing ingredient in
this ongoing debate is popular knowledge—the everyday experiences of the objects of the struggle: patients and ex-patients.
Historically, a few lone-wolf advocates have risen to promi-
nence, Clifford Beers being a notable example, but he and

others like him don't seem to have been able to make much headway. Now, substantial numbers of people calling themselves consumers and psychiatric survivors have entered the fray. In doing so, they are attempting to breach the perimeter of a tightly knit circle that has a long history of exclusive membership. The addition of a new set of actors in the traditional struggle over the truth highlights power and power relations in a new and bold way.

Power inequity and oppression

Dominance

Mental illness is a particularly difficult problem for society to deal with because it evokes in us a duality of feeling. On one hand, citizens pity the mentally ill and feel an obligation to care for them. On the other, they are afraid of them and feel in need of protection. Leifer (1990) concludes, as do most of the critics of psychiatry, that "the main social function of public psychiatry is to provide a mechanism for covert, extralegal social control without violating the principle of Rule of Law" (p. 249). This idea is intuitively attractive because power is often thought of in unidimensional terms—as limiting and constraining, even as an evil force that can harm us or make us do things we'd rather not. From this perspective, psychiatric power would be defined solely as *dominance*.

In his work on the theory of power, Wartenberg (1990) provides a kind of developmental history of dominance. He argues that a contest for power is, in its most basic form, a violent life-or-death struggle. One combatant proves stronger than the other and the loser dies. However, with the conquest comes the loss of the object of subjugation and, in a sense, both combatants lose, although obviously not equally. Hegel's famous essay exploring the power relationship between master and slave demonstrates that, in certain relationships, there is no need to prove who is the stronger because it is a foregone conclusion. Neither master nor slave wants to precipitate a life-or-death struggle, as the slave would lose his life and the master would lose his slave, along with the profit the slave would have produced. Hence, they remain locked in a relationship of domination and subjugation which doesn't need an ongoing show of force to maintain but does require a certain level of coercion.

The possibility of resistance is heightened where coercion exists. Revolts and rebellions often occur, and a natural progression in the process of domination is to develop a set of misunderstandings among the dominated so that they are more willing to collude with their oppressors in the maintenance of their inferior position. These misunderstandings become an ideology that rationalizes dominance, even in the eyes of the subjugated. Some examples of these ideologies are arguments that try to demonstrate that everyone benefits if one group is in charge, or that it's biologically preordained for some to be in a superior position. In this way, those who are dominant conceal the fact of their domination and lessen the possibility of costly incidents of resistance, achieving what is called hegemonic control. The unique aspect of hegemony is that it is largely invisible. Members of both dominant and subordinate groups alike are unlikely to question the control mechanisms that maintain the relationship.

Wartenberg extends these ideas further with Nietzsche's theories of valuation. A valuation is a judgement that acquires the guise of an objective truth that rules on the rightness or wrongness of certain behaviours. Under these circumstances, neither force nor coercion is essential to the maintenance of domination. Instead, it can be achieved merely through the medium of belief. When ideas become the tool by which domination is achieved, Foucault believes that the mastery attained is no longer associated with a threat of death but with a "taking charge of life" (as quoted in Wartenberg, 1990, p. 138). Honneth refers to this process as the *colonization* of the life-world, and describes it as "the denial of meaning, feeling, identity, individual autonomy and the appropriation and commodification of the behavioral structures of individuals" (as quoted in Gadacz, 1994, p. 111). However, ideas have little power in and of themselves without the endorsement of a higher authority. For example, the church has ruled over the powerful and the powerless alike by invoking the word of God. And, as the history of psychiatry points out, the power of God can be replaced by the authority of science.

Gil (1996) argues that the mechanisms of dominance have created a society that is structurally violent. Under these circumstances, a few are able to meet most of their needs while many may not be able to obtain even the basics of life. The result is a division where one relatively narrowly defined group occupies space within society's *universe of obligation* while others remain outside (Gamson, 1995). Gil (1996) calls this circumstance *initiating social violence* although it has many other names: subjugation, oppression, racism, sexism, homophobia, colonization and marginalization. The resulting latent energy created by oppression can foster instances of *reactive counter-violence* (rebellions, uprising, revolts and strikes) which, in their turn, are met with the meta-forces of a sanctioned and often legislated *socially repressive violent response*. The interactive spiral of initiating social violence, reactive counter-violence and sanctioned retaliation are the components of the structurally violent society in which the mental health system is embedded.

The power of those who rest inside the universe of obligation depends on a type of social "shell" that surrounds them (Wartenberg, 1990). This shell is constructed from valuations backed by higher authority, sometimes called legitimizing symbols. In the specific case of psychiatrists and other mental health professionals, an important legitimizing symbol is the acquisition of one or more formal university degrees, but it is also highly likely that they "wear" other social cues of status such as being white, being Canadian-born, being male, being straight, being middle or upper class or being wealthy. The more high status cues, the more prestigious and unassailable the social shell, and the more secure the membership within the universe of obligation. Should anyone have the temerity to question the wearer's authority, protest can be quelled through an invocation of ideas of valuation: rational scientific "truths," which are produced and maintained by the professionals themselves and backed up by what Cohen (1985) calls the higher authority of "doing good" (p. 114).

Viewed from the angle of dominance, psychiatry can indeed be construed as a power relationship that results in social control. Legitimized by the acquisition of professional

credentials, backed by the power of scientific authority and supported by an ideology of doing good, psychiatrists, as members
of the universe of obligation, have been accorded the power
under current Rule of Law to hold their patients in a psychiatric
hospital against their will for a specified period of time. Also, in
specific cases, they can force medications, seclusion, mechanical restraint or electro-convulsive therapy (ECT) upon them.
The focus of these sorts of dominant power relationships is
control of the other. The goal is compliance. The tactics used
escalate from persuasion to force and coercion. In service of
hegemonic control, such measures are called "help," and are
seen as for the patient's "own good." From Gil's (1996) viewpoint, psychiatry's role would be characterized as the maintenance of one of society's legally sanctioned repressive responses.

For your own good

Political oppression is intimately linked to psychological oppression (Prilleltensky & Gonick, 1996), meaning that the
mechanisms of dominance and subjugation can be learned very
early in life, so that they become an integral part of our view of
self. In a series of controversial books (1981, 1983, 1984), Alice
Miller charges that our Western child-rearing techniques are
inherently hurtful, coercive, humiliating and often violent—the
same criticisms that are often levelled at psychiatric treatment.

Miller hypothesizes that children, who are wholly dependent on adults for everything in their little lives, often experience parental power as dangerous, absolute, unassailable and
thwarting of their needs. In the worst-case scenario, they see
themselves as completely powerless, unable to communicate
their needs effectively or express the sense of injustice they feel
when subjected to time-honoured punishment practices (love
withdrawal, spanking, threats, shaming, humiliation, teasing,
isolation and withholding favourite objects). Expressions of
rage lead only to retaliation until the child learns to be "good,"
which in fact means fearing his or her own emotions and realities, and accepting the parental view of reality as the truth. In
Gil's (1996) terms, the child is experiencing the spiral of structural violence.

Miller points out that, while some parents are overtly abusive, most are not. The social reproduction of oppression need

not be blatant or traumatic (Prilleltensky & Gonick, 1996). It requires only that parents raise their children in the same fashion in which they were raised—internalizing experiences of dominance and mistreatment, denying feelings of rage and despair—and then repeating the same injustices with their own children, employing the oft-repeated phrase, "It's for your own good." Wooley (as quoted in Prilleltensky & Gonick, 1996) sums it up: "We are oppressed from without by a society which does not value us and therefore does not give priority to our needs, and we are oppressed from within because we have internalized those same attitudes towards ourselves" (p. 134).

Miller's ideas are disturbing and controversial and, as a result, not widely accepted in academic circles. Her work attempts to explain broader social relations and, although many exceptions can be found, her disquieting thesis is that, *most commonly*, children are harmed by our standard approaches to child rearing. Among the contributions she makes is, first, to sensitize us to the emotional life of the very small child and connect it to the adult that the child inevitably becomes. While, on the one hand, we seem to be able to understand that small bones are physically fragile and may shatter with one blow, on the other, we appear to be neglectful of the child's highly vulnerable emotional development. She also alerts us to the possibility that many of the discipline techniques that our culture sanctions in order to produce law-abiding citizens may actually harm children, and harm them in specific ways. They may grow up with a fear of their own emotions combined with very little confidence in their perceptions of reality. In short, they know exactly how bad it feels to be powerless, but they have had no opportunity to develop a sense of their own power. As a result, they can misuse that which they don't even know they have. The psychodynamic explanation for this misuse is called splitting off and projection (Miller, 1984). Essentially, children may split off and repress that aspect of themselves that they have learned to hate because it has led to so much pain—their feelings of vulnerability and powerlessness. Given that they have no way to communicate their self-hatred, children, as they grow into adults, act out their feelings by projecting their distrust of their own vulnerability onto others. Obviously, their own children are prime targets for this projection. Parents may not protect their powerless child as they should, but instead attack and belittle this "failure" with special venom. Also, society as a whole may retain deeply ambivalent feelings towards its more vulnerable citizens and feel very little obligation to examine the outcomes of its so-called good intentions. We have learned that it's what we say that is important, not what we do.

These discussions of parental dominance illuminate two aspects of power as demonstrated by the history of psychiatry and my own experiences of the workings of a psychiatric hospital. First, both the powerful—the elite and professional classes—and the powerless—mental patients—have learned about power from the same position, that of helpless children. As Janeway (1980) states: "*All* of us have experienced, one way or another, what it feels like to be vulnerable and helpless, and we can't unlive those moments" (p. 93). Thus, combining Alice Miller's view of parent-child interactions with Gil's (1996) concepts of initiating social violence provides an understanding of how the following two claims can both be true: Psychiatrists, mental health professionals, administrators, bureaucrats and politicians are members of our culture's dominant class. They do not experience themselves as dominators. As a result of this paradox, professional discourse on mental illness is rife with what feminists often call paternalism, but which might be more properly termed *parentalism*—"a model which includes not only control over, but also affectionate regard for [its] subjects" (Janeway, 1980, p. 95). The essence of parentalistic help is to offer charity and kindness on a case-by-case basis while reserving the right to withdraw aid or resort to abuse and cruelty if some sort of transgression arises. Transgressions can spring from three sources. First, the recipients of help may not display sufficient levels of gratitude. Second, they may fail to demonstrate benefit from the help they have received. They may not get well, do better or change. But the most frightening threat of all to the parental impulse is the potential for reactive counter-violence. A whole crowd of powerless and needy people, because of their numbers, cease to be viewed as worthy individuals and, instead, become defined as a grasping rabble who invoke buried memories of powerlessness and vulnerability in the dominant classes. From that point onward, it is no great leap to redefine specific vulnerable groups as a dangerous "they" who are in need of a sanctioned, repressive and often violent response which is called "help" and justified as being "for their own good." People who are situated in dominant positions but who do not experience themselves as powerful can quite easily define both kindness and coercion as for the "best." They can also back up either impulse with scientific truths and feel little incentive to examine the dissonance between the rhetoric of helping and their own actions. In other words, the fact that good intentions might not produce positive outcomes is overlooked.

Power as protest

Agency

While a social shell constructed of valued attributes surrounds the powerful, the mentally ill are imprisoned in a web of ideas of de-legitimation. These ideas, by definition, include a psychiatric diagnosis, but also may incorporate other cues such as being of colour, being an immigrant, being female, being gay or being poor. The more low-status cues, the more vulnerable and fragile the wearer's position. "He (or she) is reduced in our minds from a whole and usual person to a tainted, discounted one" (Goffman, 1963, p. 3). The mentally ill have acquired a stigmatized or "spoiled identity," and, in the process, become members of a category of people who exist outside the universe of obligation, objects of pity and fear, and potential candidates for having "good" done to them.

However, outsiders (also alternatively called the subjugated or the oppressed) are never absolutely powerless. Even under extreme conditions of repression, they have some power or "agency," as it is sometimes called. Indeed, society is often thought of as a rigid structure (in fact, Gil uses that term) which is defined merely as a set of reified societal constraints. From this perspective, agency is defined merely as our individual attempts to get around, ward off or simply cope with these constraints. However, a more useful view of the agency-structure relationship is offered by Giddens (as cited in Archer, 1990). Here, structure is defined as a set of rules and resources where only one part is constraint. In this context, agency becomes the extent to which knowledgeable human beings selectively follow the rules and use the resources that structure offers. Thus, it becomes clear that to have no choice does not mean that there is no action. In fact, madness itself has often been described as a form of protest that challenges and disconcerts by upsetting the natural order. However, as Foucault (1965) points out, this form of rebellion is usually feeble and easily defeated.

Janeway suggests three types of options available to those who are held under totalitarian regimes. The first action that can be taken is acceptance. Complete dependence on a regime and its functionaries for the basics of life can mean that people simply acquiesce, repressing any sense of injustice before it rises to the surface and demands dangerous action. The choice of acceptance is a costly one that can result in utter defeat, creating a helpless and hopeless victim or an "institutionalized" patient (Goffman, 1961). The second possibility is to get out, leave, escape, get well, or become "normal." Janeway argues that this is a particularly difficult route to take, not because the people who are caught in such circumstances lack courage, but because they lack clarity. One of the powers of a total regime is its ability to create and maintain stability through the deadly and ensnaring combination of fear and hope—fear of their keepers' power and hope that this power may, after all, be turned to beneficial use. The third action available is "disguised disobedience" (Janeway, 1980, p. 199). Patients' protesting voices, as heard in the previous chapter, demonstrate a variety of forms of disobedience. Sometimes, after release, they write exposés of their terrible treatment while incarcerated in asylums. Others write of being ignored and neglected. One politely asked to be paid for the free labour she had contributed. Some attempt to influence the nature of psychiatric treatment by pleading for more humane conditions. I suspect, however, that the more common acts of disguised disobedience were those which I witnessed during my time in a contemporary psychiatric hospital—manipulation, trickery, verbal insults and, occasionally, physical attacks, most of which were interpreted as further signs of illness rather than the tactics of resistance.

These examples of agency can annoy and perhaps even frighten, but they are not a particularly effective way to create change. While society's outsiders may possess an intuitive understanding of how power works for the powerful, they often have no appreciation of their own strength. Outsiders, just like the more powerful insiders, learn about power from the position of helpless children. Both groups tend to define power in unidimensional terms, as limiting and thwarting, and both struggle with their own blind spots. Outsiders think of power as something that everyone but them has. Given that they experience it as dominance, they conclude that it is something they do not want and withdraw in ignorance and isolation. For example, Wolfe (1993) criticizes current-day feminism for fostering a cult of victimhood. Victim feminists, as she calls them, glory in self-sacrifice, see one woman's gain as another woman's loss and insist that all women have to "equalize downward" (p. 137) in order to be true feminists.

The powerful, who also tend to define power strictly as dominance, seek ongoing affirmation that they are not dominators. They long to be viewed as right and good and, while perhaps not always kind, nevertheless possessed of a beneficent vision that renders their motives blameless—"the meeting of ardent minds in the springtime of belief is the highest award that the powerful can receive" (Janeway, 1980, p. 162). Should they not get a reasonable supply of gratitude, they can cut themselves off from their subjects and depend solely on each other to create the rules by which they will govern. "This distancing elevates them out of the human world and out of touch with their fellows, but it does not cure them of bad dreams" (p. 94). Janeway concludes that a loss of communication between the powerful and the less powerful "opens the door to fantasy and unreal expectations for both and interferes with the capacity of society to manage itself" (p. 94).

Power as a contractual relationship

The view that psychiatrists and other mental health professionals are merely instruments of social control is simply too narrow. First, it assumes that the only form of power relationship possible is dominance—an understandable position to take given the saliency of dominant-subordinate relations in our society. Second, it ignores the idea of hegemonic control, which renders power invisible to both the powerful and the powerless alike. Ideas of social control suggest that powerful people are aware of their superior status and consciously choose to use their power in a coercive manner. The less powerful, on the other hand, are seen as mindless victims, unable to affect their fate in any way. Neither statement is true. Third, it neglects the fact that there is a relationship between the powerful and the less powerful, one in which both play a role.

Janeway defines this relationship as a kind of power contract[1] and argues that "in politics, the governed consent to be ruled in return for an ordered, competent use of power that supplies them with a reasonably safe and stable environment and this consent frees rulers to act" (p. III). She believes that both the powerful and the less powerful want this contract to work because, when it does, it produces a society that functions successfully, or, in Gil's (1996) terms, one that meets basic human needs. For example, if patients were to get real, meaningful and timely help from psychiatrists and other mental health professionals, and if, upon discharge, they were able to obtain friends, family, a home and a job, they would be highly likely to view the mental health system as successful and the power contract as functional. However, most of the time power contracts don't work, mainly, Janeway believes, because those

---

1 In fact, Janeway uses Rousseau's term, "social contract," but this phrase has a particularly contemporary meaning in Ontario. In 1993, the New Democratic Party, which was then in power, negotiated what it called a social contract with its public-sector employees and unions. The goal of the contract was to reduce wages and avoid layoffs. It was a highly controversial move. Thus, in the Ontario context, "social contract" has acquired a substantially different meaning than what Janeway intends. I have chosen to substitute "power contract" in its place to avoid confusion.

in power are isolated from their "subjects." In Foucauldian terms, they are cut off from the valuable popular knowledge that arises from the everyday experiences of those who are less powerful. Certainly, the history of psychiatry is one of dominant classes talking mainly among themselves without seeking or hearing the views of patients or ex-patients.

My experience of a psychiatric hospital seems to suggest another wrinkle that must be considered. In the hospital, there were a number of power contracts operating simultaneously. Powerful psychiatrists and mental health professionals routinely defined themselves as weak in the face of administrators, and administrators, in their turn, defined themselves as weak in the face of Ministry representatives. And while it was almost always true that the patients were the least powerful in this hierarchy of power relationships, overt violence and covert "manipulation" could momentarily alter even their lowly status. When people participate in a number of power contracts at any given time, their externally defined power status (their shell) becomes contextually defined. Depending on the situation, powerful people may not at all times be powerful, nor are powerless people at all times powerless. However, Miller makes the case that, in our culture, an internalized sense of powerlessness is a stable norm for both groups.

New social movements

Given that most power contracts do not run smoothly, rebellion is a constant threat. Janeway (1980) argues that, once the less powerful understand that the powerful value their loyalty and consent above all else, they have identified their most important protest tool—mistrust. The first step in protesting the inadequate workings of the power contract is for outsiders to begin refusing to accept how insiders have defined them and to develop their own self-generated identities. Do not aspire to be normal, she advises, for the stigmatized "break the rules by being, not by doing." Instead, "accept (and celebrate) the 'spoiled identity' in public, no matter how [you] feel about it in private" (p. 245).

However, even a large measure of mistrust coupled with the redefinition of a stigmatized identity cannot sustain protest if it is experienced in isolation from one's peers. The powerful exert an intense pressure on the less powerful to see their pain and suffering as of their own making instead of the consequence of a flaw in either the ideas and actions of the powerful or in the power contract itself. Therefore, the second step in mounting a successful protest is for those who are outside the universe of obligation to come together. The resulting sense of mutuality is emotionally rewarding and fosters a new sense of trust in oneself and one's peers.

Effective protests must, then, take a third step by developing a structure for their operation. The purpose of an organizational structure is to nurture leadership and facilitate communication so that the movement can consistently renew feelings of mutuality and translate the resulting energy into activity. It is also the organization's job to create an ideology or creed that hardens the group's emotional and intellectual commitment to the cause. Ideally, an ideology serves as a legitimizing symbol for the group's new and celebrated identity. It also provides a compass that charts the movement's course, a winnowing tool that sorts through the myriad complaints and issues it could take on, searching for priorities; finally, it offers a rudder that steers members through and around the many competing ideologies of its allies and enemies so that their destination is assured.

Goldberg (1991) adds a final but essential point. Movements must be able to take effective action. Their raison d'être is to resist or promote change, depending on ideology. In essence, they are charged with the responsibility of taking control of the present and managing the future for the organization itself, and, most especially, for the membership.

There is, in fact, an entire field of study called social movement theory which has been developed to examine the genesis, strategies and fates of protesters and their movements. The utility of this group of theories lies in its ability to locate individual experiences within the concept of collective action. In other words, it will help, as have Miller, Janeway and Wartenberg, to connect individual personal experiences to the wider arena of public politics and social change.

Historically, social movement theory grew out of studies of rebellions, revolts, uprisings and industrial conflicts (Melucci,

1989)—the collective version of reactive counter-violence of which Gil speaks. Given that the exercise of early forms of dominance often employed force, countervailing measures, in their turn, tended to be violent. Issues of concern in these formative studies were confined to analyzing the conditions that moved people to collective action in the first place, the composition of a movement's membership and the nature of the action it eventually took (Melucci, 1989). Generally speaking, social movements were seen as a form of "mob rule," and theories concerning them were heavily influenced by mass psychology (Neidhardt & Rucht, 1991). Later, as dominance itself took on more subtle forms, the mob became redefined as only one form of rebellion, making it possible to include non-violent protest in research activity (Neidhardt & Rucht, 1991). In fact, Gil (1996) credits these contemporary social movements, with their emphasis on democracy and justice rather than guns and swords, as the primary force that will eventually break the destructive violence-counter-violence spiral that characterizes our present social world. Certainly, the non-violent ideologies of Gandhi and then Martin Luther King have led, first, to martyrdom and, second, to a powerful and enduring iconography that has created a valued place for non-violent protest in democratic societies. In addition, Nelson Mandela, during his inspired leadership of post-apartheid South Africa, demonstrated that revenge does not always have to follow in the wake of a great wrong.

The 1960s offered a remarkably fertile period for the study of all sorts of social protest activities. During this time, Killian (1964) was the first to suggest that movements were not the result, but the creators of social change. Mayer (1991) points out that today the term social movement embraces a multitude of social protest and reform activities; peace, environment, anti-racism, gay and lesbian, disability and the women's movement are just a few examples.

Contemporary protest has become part of the fabric of social life. Melucci (1989) argues that one of the hallmarks of these new sorts of movements is that members understand that symbolic change (often in the form of language) is an important precursor to real change. Second, they seek to make power visible. Thus, a clear understanding of the mechanisms and the uses of power becomes essential to the change process. Also, as Foucault states:

> the main objective of these struggles is to attack not so much . . . an institution or power, or elite, or class, but rather a technique, a form of power. . . . They are in opposition to the effects of power which are linked to knowledge, competence, and qualifications: struggles against the privileges of knowledge. But they are also in opposition against secrecy, deformation and mystifying representations imposed on people. . . . What is questioned is the way in which knowledge circulates and functions, its relations to power. In short, the regime du savoir. (as quoted in Plotke, 1995, p. 116)

Finally, Melucci believes that these new movements don't separate individual change from collective action. Instead, members see their own individual transformation as integral to wider societal change. In other words, they make the personal political.

Plotke (1995) argues that the older forms of social movements aimed to capture political power and redirect it in a way that was more favourable to their collectivity. New movements, on the other hand, are interested in individual power and how its exercise can positively affect their relationship to the world or, as Gadacz (1994) would argue, in breaking the bonds of their colonized internal life-worlds so that they can participate in society as fully recognized and contributing citizens. In Janeway's terms, they want a power contract that works for everyone.

Berger (1977)—an author who is not typically considered a social movement scholar—provides an avenue for the reconnection of these ideas and theories to Janeway's prescription for effective power contracts. He argues that one of the casualties of modernity has been our formally sanctioned "mediation structures . . . institutions which stand between the individual in his (or her) private sphere and the larger institutions of the public sphere" (p. 132). Much as Janeway (1980) has argued, Berger believes that modern society divides social life into the hugely public sphere—government, multinational corporations and unions, for example—and the small, private world of the individual. As a result, people feel alienated, in the Marxian sense of the word, and left on their own. Mega-structures, on the other hand, are cut off from those values and beliefs that people hold dear—Berger calls it the general morality, Foucault calls it popular knowledge—which must be understood if the powerful are to rule without resorting to coercion. He concludes his argument with two cardinal rules for the production of humane and meaningful public policy. First, it "should protect and foster mediating structures (and second), wherever possible, public policy should utilize the mediating structures as its agents" (p. 138). In Berger's terms, a protest movement is an example of an informally produced, grass-roots version of a mediating structure.

The advent of new forms of social movements is portentous. Historically, the industrial revolution transformed society's use of power by making it more efficient, less violent and orienting it toward capturing the mind instead of merely the body (Foucault, 1977). Janeway (1980) believes that "the position of the weak [has always been] a barometer of change" (p. 3) while Gil (1996) insists that these new, non-violent forms of protest are the key to changing our structurally violent society. Alvin Toffler (1990), as a contemporary prophet of social change, believes that we have indeed begun another massive "powershift," one that will affect us all. As with the industrial revolution, this period of change will not only transfer power but also transform it. The cause of the present powershift is the global availability of information and knowledge heretofore controlled and rationed by the powerful. The explosion of communication technology has meant the involvement of many more people in the production, consumption and criticism of society's erudite knowledge—its "truths." As knowledge is redistributed, so is power. Also, what is done with knowledge, once it has been acquired, is different. Previously, subjugated groups sought knowledge in order to persuade those in power to treat them fairly and more humanely. Today, with relative ease, we acquire vast amounts of knowledge whether or not we are actively seeking it and we employ this knowledge in order to become a society of "prosumers" (Toffler, 1990). Prosumerism is the fusion of consumption and production, whereby people bypass the traditional exchange economy developed as a result of the industrial revolution and develop "do-it-yourself" solutions to their own problems. Self-help is an example of pro-sumerism at work in the health care field. In case we are inclined to minimize the importance of self-help, Toffler (1990) argues that it represents a fundamental shift in our self-concept and in the nature of the professional-client power contract. While new social movements attack the regime du savoir, as Foucault terms it, the regime is itself on a path towards change. Present-day protesters are protesting different things in different ways because society itself is different.

Personal empowerment and social action

Members of new social movements appear to be struggling towards a fundamental redefinition of the power contract and of power itself—not just with simply improving on the way things are. They not only want a power contract that works, they want a contract that is different in two important ways. First, their very presence as participants in a contemporary social movement is indicative of a newly recognized power contract—one which is struck among one's peers, emphasizing equality. Gadacz (1994) argues that the social liberation of oppressed groups is intimately tied to this new form of power contract which he and others call empowerment. Empowerment is an individual process of self-liberation which he defines as "learning to overcome internalized expectations and attitudes of bitterness, helplessness, self-denial and alienation" (p. 104).

Whitmore (as cited in Lord & Hutchison, 1993) offers four assumptions that generally underlie empowerment: "a) individuals are assumed to understand their own needs better than anyone else and therefore should have the power to define and act upon them, b) all people possess strengths upon which they can build, c) empowerment is a lifelong endeavor, and d) personal knowledge and experience are valid" (p. 7).

Lord and Hutchison (1993) found that the process of empowerment usually begins with individuals getting angry or, more properly stated, becoming aware of their anger. In the context of their new awareness, they also have to have the opportunity to try out new behaviours and, paradoxically, the freedom to fail. Further, it is critical that they are supported by the external material resources that constitute the most basic of human needs, secure housing and an income, so that they can have at least some measure of control over their public, as well as private, selves. Finally, Lord & Hutchison insist that no one can become empowered on their own. They must have the company of their peers, who like themselves are struggling, improving, regressing and triumphing. They also need access to welcoming community environments such as self-help groups, social action organizations, churches, schools, employment, friends and family.

Watts and Abdul-Adil (as cited in Prilleltensky & Gonick, 1996) suggest that there can be an intimate connection between personal empowerment and politicization—the process of acquiring political awareness leading to social action. They postulate five stages: acritical ("individuals accept the legitimizing myths of personal blame and natural causes"); adaptive ("people try to adapt and benefit from whatever the system can offer"); pre-critical ("acknowledgement of power differentials but the social structure is perceived as immutable"); critical ("realization of the sources of oppression, accompanied by the impulse to work towards social change"); and, finally, liberation ("involvement in political action to eradicate personal and social injustice") (p. 139).

Gadacz concludes that

> Empowerment as a developmental and transformative process is at the heart of a social movement. . . . Reform and equality can only be pursued by empowered individuals who have learned and acquired action skills that enable them to play an ever-more conscious and assertive role in constructing their own social and political environments." (1994, p. 95)

When things go wrong

The road to liberation is not a smooth one. Internalized oppression renders revolutionaries vulnerable to reproducing both the mechanisms and discourses of domination within their own ranks. Exclusion and rejection are the de facto hallmarks of group membership along with "the attractiveness of

dogma, the temptation of certainty, the urge to control others"
(Leonard, 1994, p. 19). In addition to these destabilizing internal threats, movements can be assailed from without. Goldberg
(1991) outlines three unhappy fates that can befall them. First,
they can have no effect whatsoever, with the powerful completely ignoring their leadership and members. Second, they
can be pre-empted, meaning that their language is appropriated but real change never occurs. Finally, a movement can be
co-opted, its leadership absorbed into the ranks of the powerful
while the general membership remains in much the same state
as before. These outcomes serve as a reminder that protesters
are never guaranteed success. In fact, Gamson (as cited in
Goldberg, 1991) has found that, while approximately 40% of
movements achieve their goals, another 40% never get anywhere and the final 20% are either pre-empted or co-opted.

In conclusion

The discussions contained in this chapter make it
possible for me to talk about power, which is rarely employed as
overt analytic currency but which is, nevertheless, the disguised
subtext of mental health discourse. It also gives weight to the
necessity of examining the "other" voice in the power contract,
which has heretofore been neglected. Further, it allows me to
look at professional-client/patient and government-consumer/
survivor relationships in terms of mutually constructed, contex-
tualized power contracts instead of the traditional approach,
which tends to de-link dominant and subjugated groups and
define their activities as merely a series of opaque, unilateral
and temporally unanchored actions. Finally, an understanding
of power and power relationships connects the personal and
private experiences of early childhood, family life, mental illness, psychiatric treatment, and consumer and psychiatric
protest to the wider arena of society as a whole. It also recovers
mental patients from the deviant and pathologized margins of
social life and relocates them to a more central and main-
stream position where they are seen as both the producers and
the products of a global powershift that is affecting us all.

The questions that guide this work relate to the struggle
of consumers and survivors for liberation. They interrogate the

process of personal empowerment (how have they transformed their identities?) and connect it to social action (how have they come together collectively?). But they also reach beyond these issues, asking what happens when people join forces as a result of a common grievance. Are they able to develop a creed or organizing ideology to guide their actions? And what happens when the gaze of government, if only for a moment in time, rests upon these erstwhile outcasts, elevating their ideas and language to the exalted level of a guiding political discourse? In short, what fate awaits the consumer and psychiatric survivor movement?

4

A new power contract?

Mental health reform began over a decade ago with the publication of the Graham Report (Graham, 1988) and, although Simmons (1990) argues that most of what the document says had been said before, in fact, the authors used two new words: *consumer* and *partnership*. Toffler (1990) would argue that the appearance of these words is not particularly surprising. Along with the rest of society, health care is undergoing a powershift. Steady and reliable access to all kinds of health knowledge has led to the rise of self-help, and it has provided a nascent, but very real, way for patients to augment or circumvent traditional health care services (Levin, 1988). In addition, Immen (1996) reports that yearly up to one quarter of the Canadian population seeks treatment outside the publicly funded Medicare system, paying over one billion dollars out of their own pockets for alternative services such as herbal remedies, culturally based healing rituals, massage and acupuncture. These kinds of competitive trends, coupled with the perceived utility of attempting to apply business and marketplace solutions to the many problems Medicare faces (Rachlis & Kushner, 1994), have meant that governments and health care professionals have begun to call patients "consumers" and to formulate health policies that call for a partnership with this heretofore neglected group.

Partnership

In the context of mental health reform, the incarnation of the word *partnership* has its roots in a community mental health model called the Framework for Support (Trainor & Church, 1984). Boudreau (1990) states that this model is actually a Canadianized version of a number of American-generated service approaches that seek to redefine the community as a naturally supportive milieu. The ideological centrepiece of these models is the view that ex-mental patients are citizens and, as such, have the right to participate fully in their own communities. Boudreau adds that a further intent is to end "the imposed hegemony of professionals over the system and instead, develop cooperative linkages between the professional and the natural helping systems" (p. 9). A natural helping system is defined as those supports and resources that are commonly available in any community. Specifically, the Canadian version of the model sees clients/citizens as embedded in a four-component support network. Three of the components—self-help, family, friends and neighbours and generic community resources (such as housing and general welfare)—would be called "natural." The fourth and final component is the professional help offered by publicly funded mental health services. A further development springing from this and other like-minded models is an attempt to enhance the status of ex-mental patients by redefining them as *consumers*.

An extension of this model was the advent of the word *partnership* which, at least for a period of time, was elevated to the status of a legitimizing political symbol, called upon whenever there was a need to demonstrate unequivocally the essential rightness of a plan or policy (Boudreau, 1990). Boudreau adds that the choice of the word "partnership" was particularly powerful because it offered the illusion of "consensus and frictionless solutions" (p. 12).

However, there could be no partnership without partners. Consequently, out of the Framework for Support model arose the notion that consumer and family groups were now the legitimate recipients of governments funds, which would allow them to develop their own advocacy and self-help groups (Trainor et al., 1992). Indeed, these groups might be seen as a version of what Berger (1977) calls mediating structures, available as a utilitarian bridge between the small local world of the individual and the meta-institution of government. In fact, the Ontario government began a process of tacit endorsement of a concept called *participation*, whereby all types of institutional and community mental health services were urged to recruit consumers as members of their boards of directors, committees and task forces. The stated intention of participation, in terms of the theoretical context of this work, was to create a new form of power contract between government and consumers. However, Boudreau (1990) argues that it could also be interpreted as a logical governmental response to some extremely difficult problems. As she sees it, these problems are fourfold: "1) the exhaustion of resources and allocation of losses; 2) the loss of faith in government and the consequent need to redefine the role of the State; 3) the loss of faith in professional knowledge and professional dominance; 4) the problem of overload in a pluralist and competitive democracy" (p. 12). These difficulties add up to the perception that it may be the government's fault that Ontario citizens are paying for an expensive mental health system that is not working. And it had better do something about it.

The promise of partnership was its potential to admit consumers into the inner circle of political decision making. However, in the midst of this seemingly good-willed plan was the reality that the government is the sole funder and, in some cases, still the direct employer of all sorts of expensive medical and non-medical mental health professionals who make their living by being depended upon. These professionals were well aware that their most dominant "partner" was government and were sharp-eyed when it came to spotting a hidden agenda. At the time, Hutchison, Lord and Osbourne-Way (1986) anticipated resistance to the call to partnership, and discussed the types of excuses mental health professionals might use to suppress or avoid real consumer participation.

"They don't understand the technical language involved."

"Our clients are happy the way things are."

"We have no guidelines."

"The clients aren't motivated." (pp. 12-13)

They also identified a level of surprised scepticism among consumers, the supposed beneficiaries of the new partnership agenda:

"Our involvement has not been encouraged in the past, so we wonder why they want our involvement now."

"We are afraid that if we speak out and push for changes, they might find some way of getting back at us." (p. 11)

Barriers and excuses aside, these authors insisted that the transformative potential of partnership far outweighed its drawbacks. They argued that participation, aside from being the right of every citizen, offered consumers greater self-respect and dignity and mental health professionals new insights into old problems.

Another group of partners

Adding to the complexity of the mental health reform process was a second set of partners—the families of mentally ill people who had themselves begun to develop self-help groups combined with political activism. In Ontario, there are several formally organized family groups: the Schizophrenia Society of Ontario, the Mood Disorders Association and the Family Association for Mental Health Everywhere (FAME).

Families often have an agenda for change that is in direct opposition to the concerns raised by consumers and survivors, but the incompatibility of their respective viewpoints was not raised in official government policy. Families contend that not only do they have to deal with their relative's devastating illness and the social stigma that accompanies it but attempts to get appropriate help are thwarted by a mental health system which they argue, like other critics, is unplanned, unco-ordinated and unaccountable. They also feel that mental health professionals are trained in family-blaming treatment modalities and exhibit hostile attitudes that engender alienation and guilt (McLean, 1990). They point out that, paradoxically, these same blaming clinicians discharge an estimated 72% of their patients back to their families (Marcus, as cited in Boydell, 1996) and then when problems arise, tell them to "kick their relative out of the house" instead of offering help. In Ontario, families provide 60% of community care (Quality of Care Coalition, 1993) and, in Canada at any given time, approximately 80,000 people with schizophrenia live with their families (Seeman, as cited in Boydell, 1996).

Families state that they are not equipped to deal with mental illness and are desperate for information: what has their relative been diagnosed with? or what are the medications expected to do? Others feel that very real concerns for their own physical safety are completely ignored when their ill relative, known to have been assaultive in the past, is discharged from hospital without warning. While it remains true that most people with a diagnosis of mental illness are not violent, those who do assault often target family members (Arboleda-Florez, Holley & Crisanti, 1996; Monahan & Arnold, 1996). In fact, the level of violence towards family caregivers may be higher than previously suspected. In 1986, the National Alliance for the Mentally Ill (NAMI), an influential American family organization, sponsored a survey which found that 38% of families reported that their ill relative had been assaultive in the home at least some of the time (Torrey, 1995). However, in a recent study of Toronto mothers who were caring for sons or daughters with schizophrenia, 23 of the 25 respondents (92%) revealed that they had been assaulted by their adult child (Boydell, 1996). This researcher argues that societal norms assign caregiving functions almost exclusively to women and, as a result, it is mothers who are most at risk. Additionally, suicide is a constant and realistic fear for families. Torrey (1995) reports that from 10% to 13% of people with schizophrenia kill themselves and from 15% to 17% of people with manic-depressive disorder or depression eventually die by suicide.

Experiences such as these have led families to argue that it is really *they* who have borne the brunt of deinstitutionalization (Isaac & Armat, 1990). Weighed down by the financial, legal and emotional burdens that can accompany caring for their loved one, families often state that they need help and support almost as much as their relative (Everett, 1994b). In addition, they want mental health professionals to understand that often they are not just one of three forms of "natural" supports suggested by the Framework for Support. Mostly, they are the *only* support. Some go further, believing that government, as a cost-cutting measure, has simply shifted the burden of care from the institution to the family which, as Boydell (1996) points out, usually means exploiting the unpaid labour of women caregivers.

Finally, as a resistance strategy against blaming and stigma, most family groups are fervent supporters of the nature side of the nature-nurture debate. For example, in the United States, NAMI has lobbied for schizophrenia to be reclassified as a neurological disorder, hoping that more funds would be made available for biological and genetic research (McLean, 1990). Members of this group insist that mental illness is exclusively a brain disease and has nothing whatsoever to do with environmental or family factors. They feel that they and their ill relative should be treated no differently than when a physical illness strikes. However, Boydell (1996) discovered that viewing mental illness as a neurological disorder was not the comfort it is supposed to be. The mothers in her study constantly questioned themselves about whether or not there was "something they could have done, should have done differently" (p. 127). They wondered if their child's problem had been caused by some sort of abnormality during pregnancy, a childhood illness, violence in the home, a divorce, an inattentive father or moving to a new town. In addition, Boydell found that non-blaming attitudes on the part of mental health professionals didn't really help either. The mothers continued to feel responsible and guilty, secretly believing that if they could somehow change their own behaviour, their adult child would get well.

A public stand regarding the biological basis of mental illness and fears regarding assault and suicide have resulted in many family groups taking an advocacy position that supports involuntary psychiatric treatment. For example, some family groups have insisted on changes to the Ontario Mental Health Act because they see it as far too liberal, leading to needless deaths because families can't force their ill relatives into hospital or insist that they take their medication. In addition, some families support recent laws that allow for community treatment orders, a concept which means that certain discharged patients can be placed under a legal order where they must take their medication or else they can be returned to hospital (Boudreau & Lambert, 1993a, 1993b).

Finally, as a counter-move against the links that have been made between experiences of child abuse and subsequent mental illness (Browne & Finkelhor, 1986; Gelinas, 1983; Mullen et al., 1996; Silk et al., 1995; Steiner Crane et al., 1988), some families in Canada and the United States have founded a highly controversial organization known as the False Memory Syndrome Foundation,[1] headquartered in Philadelphia. While the group acknowledges the existence of sexual abuse, they believe that commonly quoted statistics are greatly exaggerated. They charge that irresponsible and poorly trained therapists are "creating" memories in their clients by suggesting that abuse has occurred when the clients themselves have not raised the issue (Bayin, 1993, p. 48). Indeed, in the United States, sexual abuse has increasingly become a matter for the courts as allegedly abused children charge their parents with assault, and parents, in their turn, sue therapists for creating false memory syndrome.

Given these sorts of family views and experiences, it is not surprising that their agendas for change run in opposition to those of consumers and survivors. Boudreau and Lambert (1993a, 1993b) argue that the split between family and consumer groups is based on "fundamentally incompatible discourses" (p. 80), with families most often arguing that psychiatry is helpful and no one should be deprived of its benefits while consumers and survivors usually take the viewpoint that psychiatry can be harmful and people must be protected from it. On a deeper level, these differences appear to surround the issue of power. The family side of the debate believes that society is

---

1 While non-traumatic memory may be vulnerable to suggestion, false memory syndrome is not a recognized medical condition. Studies have verified that events which children find invasive and terrorizing (such as child abuse) can be "forgotten," either because they were stored diferently in the brain or as a psychological defense mechanism, only to be recovered later in adulthood (for example, see Coons, 1994).

justified in forcing patients to accept psychiatric treatment because it's for their own good, while the consumer and survivor side insists that they have the right to refuse psychiatric treatment—even if it were for their own good—"a civil libertarian versus paternalistic or *parens patriae* conviction: the collision of views is categorical" (Boudreau & Lambert, 1993b, p. 81).

The making of policy

The making of government policy is a slow process—not incidentally because of the highly emotional sets of interests it is supposed to satisfy. In 1987, the Liberal government appointed former Canadian Mental Health Association volunteer Robert Graham to head the development of a preliminary document upon which a formal government policy statement could eventually be based. The Graham Report (Graham, 1988) heralded the beginning of a new approach to policy making. Indeed, the members of the committee that developed the report actively sought the views of their new partners—consumers and families—through a series of regional consultations. The committee also received 152 written submissions. In a study of a parallel consultation process, Church (1993) reported some of the tensions inherent in the troubled new partnership:

A professional speaks:

> We were yelled at. I remember [a person] shouting from the back of the room: "We are going to make you people hear us. Don't ever forget it. Damn it!" . . . And I went to bed that night and I was very upset. I couldn't sleep in the hotel. Because I did not come to work on these things to be yelled at. (p. 212)

Another adds:

> They were allowed to stomp out of the room. They were allowed to tell us we were assholes. . . . There were occasions when you would have liked to tell [them] off. (p. 215)

Consumers and survivors responded with:

> I don't have much sympathy for professional sensibilities. . . . Our guys are starving and dying and these guys have hurt feelings. It's really hard to swallow. (p. 226)

Clearly, the new partnership was creating a different atmosphere than had been typical for the production of government policy. A shift in the traditional power contract was under way.

Out of these sorts of uncomfortable, emotional, confrontative presentations, the Graham Report emerged. Given the different processes that had produced it, it might be expected that the report itself would be different, but Simmons (1990) believes that it defined the problems in the mental health system much in the same way preceding reports had. The Graham authors stated that there were no coherent mental health plans that identified who should be served, what services they should get, how these services should operate or where they should be located. The main issue, they said, was that there were wide regional disparities in service provision and, where services existed, there were "gaps."

The solutions offered highlighted a number of words. *Planning* was by far the most heavily emphasized requirement of a reformed mental health system. The Ministry of Health, the provincial psychiatric hospitals and the District Health Councils all needed to develop plans, and they required funds to support themselves in these activities. Also, the plans had to be multiyear and multilayered (provincial, regional and local).

A second important concept in the Graham Report was *community focused*. This idea meant that programs, whether delivered through hospitals or through community mental health agencies, had to embrace a community philosophy, meaning they had to be less illness-oriented and more dedicated to broader health determinants such as housing, financial supports, education and work readiness. The Graham Report also defined precisely which functions (rather than which programs) must be included in a complete mental health system: identification, treatment and crisis support, consultation, co-ordination, residential support, case co-ordination and case management, social support, vocational support, self-help/peer support, family support and advocacy. In order to provide these functions, the authors called for a greatly enhanced community mental health system, with funding and standards to be regulated through legislation—legislation that would have to be drafted as none existed. It also suggested training for everyone, but especially for psychiatrists, so that they could prepare themselves for roles in a community-focused system.

The third set of words emphasized by the report was *seriously mentally ill*. Serious mental illness was defined according to what are called the three D's: diagnosis, disability and duration. Naming the "target" population is a practical beginning point of many policies or reports because the size of government's fiscal obligation is dependent upon exactly how many people are entitled to its services (Simmons, 1990). However, another major factor in this decision was the clear message that this group of people has been neglected by previous attempts at reform. In addition to the severely mentally ill, several special needs groups were identified in an attempt to acknowledge the diversity of Ontario's population, endorsing at least indirectly the belief that people's gender, ethnicity, race and age affect their mental health—a view that, again, is typical of an emphasis on broader health determinants.

Next, the report emphasized the word *local*, and in this way it is very much like its predecessors. The Dymond et al. (1959), Tyhurst et al. (1963) and Heseltine (1983) reports each recommended that mental health services should be decentralized and made available throughout the province so that people could have access to help no matter where they lived. However, Ontario has what the Graham Report defines as a "rural/urban dilemma" (Graham, 1988, p. 25)—extremely densely populated areas along its southern borders coupled with vast northern regions that are sparsely inhabited. Providing services under these conditions is extremely difficult. Thus, the report also highlighted the words *coordinated*, *integrated* and *accountable*, indicating that the government needed some sort of a management strategy so that it could oversee the expenditure of its money in the proposed decentralized, and much-expanded, community mental health system.

The final word mentioned by the Graham Report was *partnership*. The report's recommendations were to be accomplished through a partnership among consumers, their families, service providers and government, although the authors were mute as to how this partnership was to be fostered or implemented.

The Graham Report was a curious blend of less government, favouring self-help and informal supports, and more government, layering on new bureaucratic structures to counteract regional disparities and to ensure co-ordination and accountability of the formal service network. The explanation for this seeming paradox lies in the fact that the report was written in a time of altering attitudes combined with a booming economy—a time when it appeared that all things were possible. It also heralded a new and powerful emphasis on the bureaucratic lens which, in contrast to the medical viewpoint, tends to see things in terms of administration and management.

Shortly after the publication of the Graham Report, the Ontario economy came to a grinding halt, plunging this perennially prosperous province into a deep and long-lasting recession. The cadillac system designed by the authors slipped further and further from grasp and many of its deadlines for implementation passed. This is not to say that *nothing* was done—far from it. In one form or another, extensive planning for mental health reform, involving hundreds of mental health professionals, consumers, psychiatric survivors, families and many, many others, has been underway since the report's publication.

In 1993, the government released its formal policy document, *Putting People First: The Reform of Mental Health Services in Ontario*, which, although ostensibly based on the Graham Report and the legislative hearings it spawned (Nelson, Lord & Ochocka, 1996), migrated considerably in both its tone and content, supposedly in response to the new fiscal reality. It also used a new term for consumers, referring to them as *consumer/survivors* (Reville & Church, 1990) in deference to the development of a more vociferous and radical branch of activists calling themselves psychiatric survivors. The notion that the government was prepared officially to call the recipients of its own services *survivors* was greeted with anger in medical quarters. Psychiatrists stated:

> The term "consumer" implies caveat emptor and, accordingly, makes no accommodation to the legal and ethical relationship of doctor-patient. By accepting this descrip-

tion, the Ministry would seem to be abandoning the relationship of trust that society has evolved in the general
interest of professionally based patient care and confiden-
tiality. The term "consumer" lowers the relationship to
that of the marketplace and serves to weaken the Ministry's case that its policy is aimed at "putting people
first." Using the term "survivor" denigrates the services
provided by professionals in the health care field. (OPDPS,
1994, pp. 7-8)

In *Putting People First*, the problems with the mental
health system were redefined in light of recessionary trends
and a perceived decline in the tax base. Expansion of the system was out of the question because the province was now
grappling with overall health care reform in response to the
sorts of pressures that began this chapter. The policy's authors
concluded that existing fiscal resources needed to be redistributed as many mental health programs were providing the
wrong type of service to the wrong people in the wrong location. As a result, an important word in *Putting People First* was
reallocation, defined as ensuring that "whenever funding and
patients are moved from institutions into the community, the
workers who provide direct care will have the opportunity to
move with the services and work in the community" (1993,
p. 27). In order to accomplish what, in essence, is a reallocation
of jobs, the policy called for a "comprehensive human
resources strategy" (p. 14), but does not offer further details. It
did, however, specify a time line; mental health reform will be
concluded by the year 2003 when one half of the psychiatric
hospital beds in Ontario will have been eliminated and an
enhanced network of community services will be in place. In
the process, the present configuration of 60% of funding for
institutions versus 40% for community programs will be exactly
reversed, creating a *balanced* mental health system.

A second problem with the mental health system, the policy stated, is its four solitudes: the psychiatric hospitals, psychiatric wards of general hospitals and other specialty psychiatric
hospitals, community mental health programs and fee-for-
service physicians. The authors argued that these four solitudes
had created an unmanageable maze where both duplications

and gaps in service were common. Thus, another word that figured prominently in *Putting People First* is *system*. The policy called for new linkages among the four solitudes that would create a co-ordinated and integrated continuum of care. And, in deference to *cost-effective*, another new concept that *Putting People First* introduced, the establishment of new mental health services were to be confined to just four elements (as opposed to the Graham Report's II "functions"): case management, 24-hour crisis intervention, housing and supports and programs run by consumers, survivors and family members. The last element referred to a concrete demonstration of the government's commitment to its new consumer partners—a program called the Consumer/Survivor Development Initiative which, in 1991, received 3.1 million dollars to develop self-help and economic development projects run for and by consumers and psychiatric survivors.

However, by far the most important word in *Putting People First* was *manage*. The policy stated that the Ministry of Health intended to take a new role as "system manager" (1993, p. 20) so that its many institutional and community programs were linked, co-ordinated, integrated, cost-effective and accountable. The new management ideology also promised to eliminate duplications, deal with gaps and generally sort things out so that the new system would begin to run with clocklike precision.

There is, however, a word that was conspicuous because of its absence. Nowhere was the term *partnership* mentioned. Consumers and their families were invited to be "involved" (p. 9) and "help" (p. 13), but their new-found status as "partners" seemed either to be irrelevant or else it was so self-evident as to no longer require official acknowledgement.

The forgotten partners

Putting People First was not well received by the government's traditional—and now seemingly former—partners, psychiatrists, hospital workers and the 10,000 unionized staff of the provincial psychiatric hospitals represented by the Ontario Public Service Employees Union (OPSEU). The authors of the policy stated that, this time, mental health reform would work because the professionals in the system were committed to co-operating with the proposed changes. This statement was true, from one perspective. *Putting People First* was soundly endorsed by the community mental health sector through the medium of this group's provincial association, the Ontario Federation of Community Mental Health and Addictions Programs.[2] The policy, at least in surface intent, implied that these services were to be the favoured recipients of the new funding reallocation strategies, engendering entrepreneurlike visions of expansion previously considered only a dream. Thus, community mental health professionals were not necessarily concerned with a close scrutiny of the policy, having concluded that their battle for recognition was over and won.

However, psychiatrists and physicians were livid. They argued that mental health reform meant job loss, pure and simple, and insisted that, without an attendant massive retraining strategy coupled with transitional funding, co-operation from the medical community would be highly unlikely (OPDPS, 1994). In a strong "hell-no-we-won't-go" message, unionized workers added that community mental health agencies, which were supposed to become the new employers of reallocated institutional staff, were rarely unionized themselves, were notoriously underfunded and offered benefits and working conditions inferior to those of public service employees (OPSEU, 1991). In addition, they pointed out that *Putting People First* didn't even mention the cavernous 25% wage gap between institutional and community workers.

Putting People First argued that reform plans were based on an extensive process of consultation with consumer/survivors and their families. Physicians and psychiatrists argued that the use of the term consumer/survivor was insulting and, while not opposing patient or family involvement in principle, they decried the lack of acknowledgement for the fact that institutional staff were also partners. They insisted that the Ministry's policy had created a false dichotomy—an institutional-versus-community atmosphere which contributed directly to

---

2 I was a member of the Board of Directors of this organization during this period, and thus bear personal witness to these claims.

the four solitudes it criticized. The union added that *Putting People First* was simply a plan for expenditure control. Under mental health reform, they predicted, provincial psychiatric hospitals will become nothing more than "warehouses for the severely ill and jails for dangerous patients" (Dukzsta, as quoted in OPSEU, 1994, p. 7).

The policy also stated that mental health reform would work because the Ministry of Health had extensively studied experiences in other jurisdictions and, as a result, developed a plan that was solidly built upon what they had learned. The physicians countered that the ideas the policy proposed were "more a matter of applied political skill than of mental health requirements" (1993, p. 4). They added that what other jurisdictions had actually discovered was that closing psychiatric hospitals had resulted in a large increase in the homeless mentally ill population. Families joined the physicians in this latter concern, believing that a decreased role for hospitals and institutions would mean that their relatives wouldn't be able to get the help they needed when they experienced crises (Beeby, as quoted in OPSEU, 1994).

Further, according to *Putting People First*, an important key to the success of reform was to build on existing effective community programs. Physicians argued that community agencies had neither the expertise nor the desire to handle the needs of the seriously mentally ill. The union added that community mental health in Ontario was a euphemism for "underfunded, under-staffed and over-burdened services struggling to cope with growing caseloads on shoe-string budgets" (OPSEU, 1991, p. 2). Inadequate budgets meant low staff salaries, which translated directly into poor quality of care for patients and clients. Both groups agreed, and were supported in their views by independent policy analysts (MacNaughton, 1992), that community programs had to be beefed up *before* institutions and hospitals were downsized or else there would simply be a repeat of the many ills associated with deinstitutionalization in the 1970s.

Finally, the policy stated that mental health reform would work because it was based on realistic goals and time lines. Physicians and psychiatrists insisted that *Putting People First* was essentially a document for administrators. It talked in terms of budgets and beds per hundred thousand and neglected the real issues, like treatment and the roles of health care professionals. They concluded that the policy was simply a prescription for pulling precious funds from direct service delivery in favour of layering on expensive bureaucratic structures, reflecting an entirely self-serving attitude on the part of the bureaucrats who penned the policy in the first place. These critics believed that *Putting People First* demonstrated all too clearly exactly which people it intended to put first.

In conclusion

The context for the rise of consumer and psychiatric survivor activism was the period of mental health reform as defined by the Graham Report and *Putting People First*. The stated intention of recruiting "consumer/survivors" as partners was the creation of an improved mental health system where people could get appropriate help, when and where they needed it. However, physicians and unionized hospital workers argued that this new partnership had been formed at their expense and that its goal of creating a cost-effective, balanced and well-managed mental health system was, in reality, a thinly disguised justification for job loss and layoffs for workers with a concomitant rise in status of bureaucrats and administrators. This dialogue and these actors set the stage for the many stories and struggles that I report in the following chapters.

5

A special bond

Mental patients and ex-mental patients are a diverse group of people. Among them, they represent all the variations that are characteristic of the whole population of Ontario. Yet, they are finding their way to one another, forming small groups in their respective communities and then attempting to merge these groups into a larger collectivity. When they meet, they recognize "some common basis of life" (Simmel, quoted in Levin, 1971, p. 11) which makes them, at one and the same time, similar to one another and different from other categories of people. They say they have a "bond" that is unique and not shared with any other group (Oswin, in *OPSAnews #1*, 1990, p. 6). In Simmel's terms, they impose upon one another a veil of mutuality that obscures individual differences and creates a sense of fusion. They are attempting to meld their seemingly individual voices into a shared cry of protest.

Telling stories

In my research, the specific question that turned out to be an entree into this topic was: "What forces led to your original involvement in the psychiatric system? What did you expect and what did you get?" I originally formulated the question as a way of talking about the types of life problems and difficulties that precipitate admissions to psychiatric hospitals. My own experience had been that there seemed to be no single route patients followed that led inevitably to the doors of a hospital. Instead, a series of factors, many of which appeared external to the person, seemed to pile one upon the other, culminating in some sort of behavioural outburst that the individuals themselves, the police, family or neighbours thought best defined in psychiatric terms.

In the interviews, I usually followed this question with a prompt intended to emphasize that I was asking about the *forces* respondents thought led to psychiatric hospital admissions, which they may or may not wish to illustrate with personal information. From my own past experience, I understood that events that precipitate admissions to hospitals are often embarrassing or painful to recall. I wanted respondents to be free to focus on the "big picture" if they wished, instead of feeling cornered into revealing private material that they would rather leave undisclosed.

The second part of the question (What did you expect and what did you get?) was designed to get a sense of what expectations respondents had when they asked for help from the mental health system (usually a psychiatric facility). I also wanted to know whether or not they felt these expectations had been met. Obviously, I harboured an a priori opinion, developed as a result of my experience as an inpatient psychiatric social worker. I believed that, as professionals, we'd promised a lot but failed to deliver, and frankly I did not expect to hear accounts of satisfaction. The underlying purpose of this question was to develop a catalogue of respondent-defined life difficulties that led to a request for help, accompanied by a corresponding set of assessments as to why help was not forthcoming.

Respondents answered the questions, not with an objective, intellectualized discussion of precipitating forces or an inventory of complaints—the "big picture" I was expecting—but with intensely personal stories that, in essence, were their version of their own history. They began to provide the answer to the first question I had posed, when I asked by what process they had come to reconstitute their identities. Of course, the whole of each interview was a "story" in the broadest sense of the word, but these questions elicited a unique kind of story-within-a-story, which was typically lengthy, told without pause and with great passion. It tended to proceed in sequence, with a beginning, middle and end. Kohler Riessman (1993) speaks of narrative styles where tellers "pour their ordinary lives into archetypal forms" (p. 19). If this is the case, then these are odysseys where struggling heroes embark upon dangerous journeys through inhospitable lands, encountering villains along the way before arriving at their destination, wiser but also sadder because they have learned a hard lesson and paid a heavy price. The stories are historical in the sense that they speak of real people and report actual events; however, they must be understood, not as objective facts, but as representations of them. As a final comment, I had the sense that many of these stories had been told before, not just internally as a form of meditative dialogue, but publicly, with an audience to reflect back responses that alerted the teller to the rough spots, which were smoothed away for the next telling, until the story shone forth as a version of personal truth.

Consumers and survivors have been the objects of psychiatric history for well over two hundred years, their lives and experiences appropriated and defined by supposedly well-intentioned others. However, Flack (as quoted in Gamson, 1991, p. 47) argues that "people are capable of and ought to be making their own history." Personal histories are "made" through storytelling where people reconnect themselves to their own account of the past so that present life becomes intelligible (Gersie & King, 1990). Freire (1970) states that it is important to "name the world" (p. 80) by placing one's own reality on life events. And, according to Malhotra Bentz (1989), this reality can be even more important than the event itself. The pursuit of objective truth, at least in the scientific sense, is beside the point. The "truth" of narratives cannot be proved. Instead, storytellers seek a representation of reality which is intimately connected to the listener and bounded by the interpretive dialectic they create together. Respondents' stories represent a metaphorical liberation as the authors re-appropriate what Gadacz (1994) calls their "colonized life-worlds." Janeway (1980) adds that it is the prerogative of the less powerful to reject how the powerful have defined them and begin to develop their own identities, which are given substance and verisimilitude through the repeated telling of stories, until both private and public expressions of the present self are recognized as congruent with past experiences and predictive of a fresh, future-oriented identity.

The following four stories are examples of recovered histories that form platforms for the development of new identities. I selected these four because the storytellers (three women and a man) are clearly very different people, but each eventually shares a similar fate—they end up on a psychiatric ward. While as a researcher I was interested in how they got there, respondents, on the other hand, were much more concerned about how they got out.

While I could have chosen to break up the stories into their components or themes, hoping for a deeper understanding of experience through partialization, in the end I decided that to do so would have done violence to their intended meaning. They represent an indivisible gestalt of experience, which requires an intact telling from beginning to end, so that their similarities and differences are allowed to emerge organically from the narrative context—as the teller intended.

Four stories

Susan Marshall lives in Fort Francis, a small town some distance from Thunder Bay in the northwest quadrant of Ontario. She has three children from her two marriages. She is divorced from her second husband and has her youngest daughter living with her. Susan is in her late thirties and is employed as the co-ordinator of a Consumer/Survivor Development Initiative self-help project located in her area.

> I was brought up in a home where the message was that we were strong people and mental illness—I don't even know that I heard the word as I was growing up—but it was definitely a no-no and if anybody suffered from any kind of problem like that, they were less than the rest of us, that's for sure. So when I started having problems, I didn't even recognize what was happening. I just knew that I was "less than" and I had to hide that. So I ended up making my problems way worse than they ever had to be because I hid

them for years and years. You know, sometimes, I didn't come out of the house for six months.

At one point, I moved to a city in Saskatchewan where I got involved with the women's movement. Somebody suggested that I go to this "nice" person that they went to for help. Well, I didn't realize what a psychiatrist was to begin with. Not at all. I didn't even realize the wide, sweeping powers they have or anything else. I was totally ignorant.

So, I ended up going to this psychiatrist and she *was* a really nice lady and I think, maybe, I was a bit lucky in that regard. She diagnosed me as manic-depressive. That was like a real "Oh my God!" kind of thing. I was put on lithium and it just wasn't working. And then she suggested that I go into hospital for a few days so they could monitor the medication. So I said, "Sure, that's OK." No big deal. I was just too dumb to know.

So I ended up trying to get off the ward at night— just innocently trying to leave. And they wouldn't let me. They wouldn't let me go and I got hysterical, which I now recognize was a completely normal response. Then things got really out of hand and I ended up being tied down. I was committed involuntarily for a few weeks and as soon as I could I left. . . . Basically what I did was I learned very quickly to play the game and I hid everything that was going on and gave the answers that were expected. Thank God, I'm intelligent enough, you know, to realize these things and I disappeared as soon as I could. Got off the ward and disappeared. And stayed back in the closet for a long, long time, too afraid to go that route again.

Jennifer Reid was 33 years old when she told me her story. I met with her in her "suite" of offices—what she jokingly called the small, slightly seedy fourth-floor walk-up location of her survivor-run drop-in program, where she is the director. She describes herself as a lesbian, part black and part Native, but *all* feminist. Adopted by a white, middle-class family as an infant, Jennifer felt that she never really belonged—"there were no roots for me." She says she's been fighting the "system" for over 15 years.

I hadn't met Jennifer before the interview and she was cordial but a little wary. She seemed to tell her story as a way of setting me straight about where she was coming from. She started by announcing her "bullshit" diagnosis—Jennifer says that psychiatrists call her a sociopath.

> I'm an incest survivor. And when I was 19 years old, I ran into a guy who reminded me of the man who abused me, and I hit him. The problem was that I didn't stop hitting him and I ended up going to prison for six years. Well, nine, but shit happens.
>
> I went into the Kingston Prison for Women and they have a case management worker who assesses you and figures out where you should go. At the time, I was having flashbacks from the abuse and I was very angry. I was upset because the traditional agencies, from the time I was 16 to the time I was 19 when I went to prison, were not LISTENING to me. And I'm talking about agencies in Brampton and hospitals in Peel and in Toronto. And I'm talking about the private school I went to. They blamed it all on a learning disability. And that's not the truth. Part of my behaviour problems might have been because of the learning disability, but another part was because of racism, and the major part was because of abuse. So I ended up in prison.
>
> My case management officer saw something was up and that it had to do with abuse, so she got a woman from Queen's University, J., who was doing her Ph.D. on sexual abuse survivors. J. and I started working on the abuse so that was basically my first contact with a psychologist. In Prison for Women, they had psychiatrists, a male and female, and their answer to everything was to give you Largactyl which, to me, is bug juice. All it did was dope me up and make me go to sleep. J. worked on the issues.
>
> Eventually, I got out of prison on a full parole, but I wasn't stable enough to be out on the street, I realize now. When you're in jail, your meals are made for you, you have a set time to get up, a set time to go to work, go to school, go to sleep. You get locked down. You have a set time to do everything. They don't give you life-skills training to handle life on the street and, after four years, it was heavy. It was hard to just adjust. So I ended up going back in.
>
> Then I got into a fight with another woman prisoner and the warden put me in segregation. A segregation cell is six feet by three feet. Twenty-four-hour fluorescent light, a steel toilet and a steel bed—locked up for twenty-three and

a half hours a day. If you're good, they might let you walk around the yard, which they called the "tennis court."

So after months of going absolutely nuts, they gave me a choice on December 19. They said, "You can either stay in segregation until after Christmas, which is the worst time of year to be locked up, or you can go to a psychiatric hospital. Now, the hospital has got green grass, Jennifer, and you'll have a nice little bed and you'll get to wear your own clothes and you'll get to listen to the music you want to listen to and you'll be able to smoke filtered cigarettes instead of roll-your-owns and you'll be able to walk around and associate with people." So I, being the innocent that I was about mental institutions, said, "OK, fine."

They took me up in the elevator and took off my handcuffs and my leg irons. And as the elevator door closed behind me and I walked down this long hall, I realized I was trapped. I was out of the correctional system and into the mental health system and the two, as far as I'm concerned, are the same.

The staff consisted of two psychiatrists, one psychologist, a social worker and nurses. Now some of the nurses were trained, but the majority of them weren't trained for psychiatry at all. They left the day-to-day workings of the ward and the groups—the social therapy side of it—to these men who ran the program. These men had killed people. They had raped women. They'd raped little boys. These men raped animals. These were the men that were teaching *me* how to become a sane person. They were the "teachers" and what that meant was they made you sit on a floor in a room for four hours and not move. And you had to hold up your one finger to ask to go to the bathroom. If the teacher didn't like you, and they didn't like me because I was mouthy and a lesbian, they made you wet yourself.

So I got pissed off, got really angry and they threw me into this room called the "side room" which is just a cell where they tie you down to a mattress. They handcuff your legs. They handcuff your hands and then they strap a sheet across your body. And if you are really "lucky," they give you a shot of Haldol and sometimes they forget to give you the side-effect drug which is Cogentin. Well, I got Haldol because I'm a borderline personality disorder, and a sociopath with psychopathic tendencies—that's how they diagnosed me. I was a sociopath because I was a lesbian, OK? And a psychopath because they decided from my tests that my hostility level was way above. Well, that sort of made sense to me considering I'd been abused and been in a prison. It also said that I was a "traditional overly dependent female," meaning that I was a heterosexual woman who was playing at being a lesbian. And they said that if I went through their treatment, I would come out of the hospital not a sociopath anymore. I would come out as a heterosexual female on her way to getting married and BE CURED! Needless to say, 10 years later, I'm still a lesbian and I'm still a sociopath and very proud of it.

The hospital was an interesting experience because you learned how to manipulate. I mean, they made me go on strip status—strip status was you had to wear their clothes—because I wouldn't wear a bra. Now, I had no chest at that time so I didn't feel I had to wear a bra. They made me write out, the very first time I got caught without a bra, 50 times, "I must wear a bra." Rule number 53. I'll never forget rule number 53 because I had to write it out 500 times after the first 50. And the men would go behind you and put their hands down your back to see if you were wearing one. Now for an incest survivor or any type of abuse victim, that would trigger something that would give them reason to keep you in longer and to medicate you and to give you shock treatment. I lasted there for two years, and then one day a friend came in to see me and said, "Jennifer, what the fuck are you doing here? You are NOT nuts."

By that point in time, I was "relating" and relating was a two-second kiss at the front door and a two-second kiss at the back door with a man. It was to get them off my lesbianism. My "date" was an incest survivor himself and he knew I was a lesbian and he was Native and I'm part Native so we both "related"—they called it relating—having a relationship. You could walk around the yard holding hands and he would pull your chair out for you and be a perfect gentleman and everything. And all it was was manipulation to get them off my back.

Anyways, I started relating and I got enough privileges that I could have a handcuff key . . . be on the security team so I could throw somebody else down and tie them to a mattress. I also got a lighter. That meant I didn't have to run around trying to get somebody to light my cigarette. I ended up sitting on their treatment committee, which was made up of a staff and other patients and we assessed new patients when they came in and assessed people every single day. I sat on the sanctions committee, which was the punishment committee. I became an assistant teacher and then a teacher. Hey, teachers got to stay up half an hour longer. So, to me, it was just straight manipulation. Was any of the borderline personality disorder dealt with? No. Was the abuse dealt with? No.

Their idea of dealing with someone was . . . there was one woman in there who was delusional. Before she came in, she was 27 floors up in her apartment and she threw her baby out of the window because she thought she was sending it to God. In the hospital, she would never go near a window and was one of the sicker patients. And we had these intense groups . . . it could go on for as long as three days, two hours in, two hours out, two hours in, two hours out. But the person that is the object of the group doesn't get to sleep. They feed them but they don't get to sleep. It's called breaking a person.

Anyway, with this woman, I saw it and that's when I started to rebel. Somebody noticed that she wouldn't go near a window 'cause she threw her baby from a window so they had a group on her by a window. They put up a blanket and held her by the window until they broke her and if anybody thinks, . . . when you transcribe this and they read this, that I'm not willing to say this to their face, they've got another think coming. I've been saying this about them for years—publicly, in the newspapers, and in videos and on the radio. That's just one case. I mean, for me, it was a little bit easier because I was just an "overly traditional female"—dependent female at that, and needed just to get away from being a lesbian. And all I did was manipulate. I related with this guy who had some of the same problems I had. We held hands, had our two-second kiss and laughed at them and I got out and he got out.

The narrator of the third story is Marilyn Nearing. I interviewed Marilyn by telephone. She lives in Keswick, a small town about one hundred kilometres north of Toronto. Marilyn is in her late forties, married and the mother of a 19-year-old son. Al-

though she was describing painful experiences, the telling of her
story was interspersed with delighted and infectious laughter.

Some years back, I was working for Revenue Canada when
my life was threatened by a disgruntled taxpayer. I had
been a person who thought that you could control your
destiny, mind over matter, and it was the first time in my
life that I had ever experienced physical illness and re-
occurring headaches. I had manoeuvred through life pretty
successfully, bowling people over. I had a survival technique
that worked for me and that meant shutting out the rest of
the world and believing that I could just wish things away.

When I first got ill, I thought it was totally physical—
high blood pressure and migraine headaches that I never
had before. I was assured—I assured myself—that I had a
brain tumour and that I was either going to die or they
were going to operate and it was going to be OK. Eventually
I started having flashbacks and re-experiencing childhood
sexual abuse. I think I'm probably one of the classic cases
of repressed memory. By then, they had got me addicted to
painkillers—*never* self-administered, I might add. I used to
get daily shots of Demerol from my doctor. I got so I could
walk and move with it and it didn't do anything. I couldn't
do without it either. I truly became addicted. So now I had
two problems. By the time that I decided that dying would
have been a better option, I was not only suffering severe
depression and chronic pain but I was also having flashbacks and wondering why I wanted to murder my brother. I
had also become virtually bedridden for the better part of
two years. Through addiction and mental health problems,
I finally realized that these little flashbacks had to mean
something and I went to a psychiatrist.

So, I was diagnosed with depression. I also managed
to go into hospital and come off Demerol which was no
easy feat. And while I was institutionalized on the local psychiatric ward, I saw how people were treated. I was just
dumbfounded. I couldn't believe it. I had come from an
omnipotent position—the tax-collector and enforcer—to
having no power and authority, and I saw people abused
even more than I was because, even at my sickest, I was
still somewhat in control. I just couldn't believe it, and I
had to re-examine my whole belief system about schizo-
phrenics and manic-depressives and clinically depressed

people. I mean, I had a real revelation. These are people that have problems and who will get well if they get support. I just couldn't believe the cesspool of discrimination that was there.

I then started into therapy about the flashbacks. It was a grueling two- or three-year process identifying the memories, having them validated. Fortunately, I got a psychiatrist who wasn't too busy at the time and could take a fair amount of time. I don't know whether his business was growing or he was incapable of dealing with it, but he referred me to a group here in York Region and also to a program for abuse issues that they had at the hospital run by an occupational therapist. Those two programs really did a lot of good for me and at least this doctor referred me and didn't sit on it. I have seen women in the system for years and years where they don't get well until the abuse issues have been dealt with. They go through the traditional mental health system, diagnosed and rediagnosed over and over again and finally someone twigs to the abuse and, like myself, they get better.

Then, of course, everything that happened in my body became psychosomatic instead of physical. I started having flooding. . . . I was having three periods a month. I mean, all I had was periods. I should have taken out shares in Kimberly Clark. It was just horrendous. And I really had difficulty getting to a female gynecologist. But I finally found one and she saw me one day when I was flooding—just like I had told everybody I did. She said, "You can't live like this." I'd already told three male gynecologists and they'd said to me, "There, there, Mrs. Nearing, it will be all right." I had a hysterectomy and I haven't had a period since. Glory hallelujah! Give me hot flashes any day.

Anyway, I realized that you cross that border one day. At first everything was physical and they would only look at me that way, and the next day it was all psychosomatic and they'd only look at me that way. It's a real struggle to get them to look at you as a whole person, you know, and deal with everything. It's when you're asked to divide yourself up in pieces—or when they divide you up for you. . . . It's no wonder we go crazy!

Paul Reeve is the final narrator. At 43 years of age, he is divorced and, at the time of the interview, was the co-ordinator of a consumer- and survivor-run program in Guelph. When I asked how he would like me to describe him, he said that all I needed to say was that "bald is beautiful." Paul's story, perhaps more than any other, emphasized the "pouring" of his life's journey into an "archetypal form" (Kohler Riessman, 1993, p. 19). He also moved beyond the boundaries of his disillusionment with psychiatry and psychiatric hospitals, and offered a description of the alternative forms of help that he eventually found.

> I remember the very first psychiatrist I went to. I'd lost my job and I was devastated. I think it's fairly typical as a male. I took a lot of my identity from my work and I was a workaholic. So I started moving into what they call a major depression. I call it deep, deep despair. And I had a psychiatrist tell me that I would have done better if I had quit my job, gotten out of my marriage and moved away from my home. And all I know was, at that time, everything in my body and my head said, "No." That's all I could say. "No, you're wrong." I can't even be sure that I even expressed that to him. I may not even have had the strength. I had expected him to tell me something that would make me be better. But, instead, I got a psychiatrist telling me what to do and the other side of the equation was I didn't get better.
>
> After six months my wife did leave. She said she didn't wish to be around someone who wasn't capable of pulling themselves up by their bootstraps and my little hummer went off again.
>
> I call it my hummer. I think the books call it a conscience or something. It hums in me. It's wonderful. If I'm in a situation now, I trust my hummer. I move when my hummer tells me to move, not when my head does.
>
> Anyway, medications were being pushed on me. "Try this medication," and I'd try it and I'd have dry mouth or my stomach would hurt or I wouldn't be able to see very clearly, lots of different body reactions. I just stopped. And they'd keep pushing more and more medication and my hummer would say, "No, no." And then they started calling me names, "You're a resistant patient. You're going to be dead because you're not listening to me. You're going to go out and kill yourself." I was suicidal at the time. It was

an option and, not seeing any other alternative, the only option.

So I think all of that helped me to eventually work towards trusting my hummer and I did seek out alternatives, almost on an unconscious level. Everything told me that I couldn't heal that way.

My belief is that whatever lessons, whatever positions we are put into in life, we'll keep returning to that until we "get it." So, when I was 17 years old, I was in a mental institution and 27 years later, bang, right back there and almost in exactly the same spot and experiencing the same situation. I even lost a girlfriend earlier and this time I lost a wife.

So it was almost as if I had to go back to see what the lessons were that I didn't get—or hadn't been offered at age 20. You see, it's hard to learn the lessons you need to as long as the mental health system keeps telling you, "We have the answer. . . . We're going to find the right drug. We're just working on these drugs—they've got some side effects but we're gonna find the ultimate one . . . real soon . . . we hope."

And what I found—I'll never forget what I found the first time I walked into a 12-step group when I was in very deep despair. I walked in and somebody just said to me, "I'm really glad you're here. And, we love you. And you don't need to do anything." And that was like, profound, and my whole recovery is based on that. All of a sudden, I got it. "I don't have to do anything and I'm OK." That's like a 180-degree shift from going to professionals and hearing them say, "We're just going to try one more medication . . . one more therapy. We've got to try this avenue. There's just SOMETHING we got to do in order for you to get better."

And here's a 12-step group, run in a little church basement and nobody had any credentials or anything other than love and acceptance. I just wept through the whole meeting. Nobody had ever said . . . boy, I get feeling sad . . . happiness and sadness right now. Somebody said, "You're OK right where you are, Paul." I began reading again and calling people and reaching out and asking what is this spiritual stuff? There was this whole new world and nobody had told me about it.

So, ultimately, my strength carried me slowly towards something that worked. I went into a chapel one day, it's called Mount Carmel. It's in Niagara Falls. I have no religious background. I don't go to church. I walked into this chapel and I was so low. Anyway, there was a priest there and I said in all sincerity, "I think I need religion because I'm losing the battle here and I'm losing it quick. I'm going down." And it was a sincere question . . . or a sincere desire because somehow there was a spark in me that didn't want to die, but I didn't have any answer.

And the priest looked at me and smiled and said, "I think religion's the *last* thing in the world you need." And I'm thinking, WHAT? My last little hope. And he said, "But if we can find a little bit of spirit in you, maybe we'll have a good start." From there on, he gave me support and encouragement and allowed me to be in the church for many months. I would go every day, and for many weeks the best I could do was go and sit . . . sit in the chapel and cry.

I cried for months. All of that was healing. I was just releasing what was frozen inside of me. To this day . . . why did I walk into that place? It's absurd. At any intellectual level, I just couldn't . . . so something inside me does take me where I need to go even when I'm not aware of what it is.

And the next thing I did, well, I ended up on a plane. I called a place on a Thursday and ended up on a plane to Texas the next Tuesday. Again, my hummer said, "Just go." I was still pretty bad and ended up with a wonderful, beautiful lady. She's a psychiatrist. She gives no medication. She is not well liked by her profession, by her peers. And she was able to say to me, "You need your feelings. You have them . . . you just need to get in touch with them." She was connected to her heart. She was able to share her experience, to be a human being with me. I got to see a human being across the desk . . . well, it wasn't across a desk . . . it was in a room. It was incredible. That was probably about the seventh psychiatrist I had been to and I finally found hope.

Sadly mistaken

Janeway (1980) believes that both the powerful and the less powerful want their power contract to be a success. "We want to believe that things are going well, that princes can be trusted to act wisely and sages to foresee the future correctly" (p. 164). Clearly, these storytellers are both sad and angry with a psychiatric power contract which they believe let them down. As Supeene (1990)—a survivor herself—writes, "They'd promised to *help* me (p. 71) and, instead, "abuse and oppression is what psychiatry meant by help, care and therapy" (p. 231). Jennifer Reid adds:

> These people are professionals. You would think they would know what they're doing, that they would help me with the abuse, that they would help me with all my issues so I'd get better . . . be able to go out into society. I believed that they would fix things. That's how I was raised. Well, I was sadly mistaken.

In addition, there is a sense of embarrassment because respondents were, as Susan Marshall says, "just too dumb to know." As a result, they see themselves as especially fortunate because getting out of a psychiatric hospital did not entail the expected path of receiving help and getting better. Instead, it involved a combination of luck and manipulation which respondents define as going along with the rules and telling professionals what they wanted to hear—"I'm fine"—when they really felt the same, or worse, as when first admitted.

In the end, a resolution for respondents' problems—"issues" as Jennifer Reid calls them—had to be found somewhere else, and good fortune was seen as the companion that guided the journey. Paul Reeve calls it following his "hummer," and many respondents, in the standard colloquial way, thanked God for their good luck.

> "Thank God, I'm intelligent enough. . . ."

> "God, if I hadn't already been familiar with the Mental Health Act. . . ."

> "If I hadn't had the social supports that I had. . . ."

"I guess I had enough stubbornness, enough stupidity, enough fight. . . ."

"I was fortunate because I slipped through the cracks. When they do their assessments, they say I resist authority . . . don't respect authority, whatever. For me, that's a redeeming feature because I never got sucked in."

McGuire (1990) believes that, in order for narratives to persuade, they must reach beyond content (the facts) and form (an odyssey), and present a moral or lesson. In this case, the hero of the story, with the supposed aid of luck, is transformed from unknowing innocent to someone who finally sees the truth. However, a close reading of each story reveals that considerably more than luck contributed to the transformation. Each teller was an active agent in his or her own redemption— observant, resourceful, persistent, creative—and courageous. Given that they perceived themselves to be in the grasp of a totalitarian regime, they chose the most difficult resistance strategy of all. They escaped.

But, as Janeway has stated, people who believe themselves to be powerless are among the least capable of accurately assessing their own strength. These are stories where a positive resolution is attributed only to forces considered outside the teller's control. God and luck, instead of individual power and agency, are the perceived guides for this set of heroes as they make their escape from danger.

In fact, respondents tended to view their exit from a psychiatric hospital or psychiatric treatment as a form of abandonment rather than liberation. Each storyteller reluctantly concluded that psychiatry's promise of help, while initially raising hope, turned out to be as cruelly empty as a desert mirage. Instead of finding the comforting and restorative haven that would end their weary journey, respondents found themselves forced back out onto a lonely road, carrying the added burden of bitter disillusionment. Perhaps, in this sense, the stories are reminiscent of the most famous odyssey of all—the biblical fall where Adam and Eve, after eating the fruit of the tree of knowledge, are banished from the garden and forced to make their way in a dangerous and uncertain world. In service of the rhetorical purpose of the narrative—to persuade and inform—

respondents seem to have built their story within a familiar framework that serves to strengthen their connection to their audience and, by extension, their argument. It is not, however, a framework that celebrates triumph and freedom. Instead, it emphasizes desertion and loss.

The stories began with a call for help which respondents believed would be answered within the bounds of the traditional psychiatric power contract. After all, the mental health system promises help and, as Jennifer says, "I believed they would fix things." However, Janeway (1980) believes that such faith is akin to believing in fairy godmothers. Scepticism and disbelief, she says, are the essential accoutrements of adulthood, creating "an autonomous creature centred in an independent self" (p. 165).

Yet, it must be acknowledged that Paul, in particular, described an extensive search for a rescuer, and his persistence finally paid off. Paul was not alone. More than a few respondents reported that they eventually found help within the mental health system, and it was provided by a mental health professional.

"J. worked on the issues."

"Those two programs really did a lot of good for me."

"I ended up with a wonderful, beautiful lady . . . she's a psychiatrist."

"I found a woman who listened to me."

"My shrink sent me to an advocacy program where I became aware of my rights."

"I found a male psychiatrist who was very helpful."

"I found a community program that made all the difference."

"I was seeing a psychiatrist and he was actually very good."

Respondents conclude that these "finds" are also lucky events, and in this Miller (1984) might concur. She argues that power relationships which encourage, teach, nurture and guide are not the common basis of our society's child-rearing practices and may indeed be rare experiences in adult life. Nevertheless, these seem to be the sorts of relationships respondents hoped for when they entered into the psychiatric power contract. In the face of dashed expectations, they speak of themselves as "sadly mistaken" and "lucky" if they actually got what they wanted. Indeed, having got what they wanted—finally—appears not to have erased memories of previous failures. They now know that things can go badly wrong for the innocent. They feel alienated and adrift—left on their own (Berger, 1977). They can see what others do not, and the process by which that knowledge was acquired was deeply disturbing—in fact, traumatizing may not be too large a word to describe how they feel about it.

A special bond

Powerless people are especially aware of their own vulnerability if power contracts fail because they are the ones most likely to suffer. When things turn out badly, stories are a valued method for making sense out of the trauma. The construction of a story is, in fact, an achievement, which first connects emotion to experience and second scans the inner and outer life-world in order to develop a causal chain of events that establishes meaning (Wigren, 1994). It draws conclusions that are intended to create an understanding of what happened. Stories also constitute an essential part of human interaction as people connect to one another through the telling and retelling of their personal histories. Mutual understanding, according to Bruner (1995), "assumes social obligations of the most binding and serious kind" (p. 27). In other words, it creates a special bond, one of the necessary precursors to mounting a successful protest (Janeway, 1980). As an example, this brief fifth story demonstrates that it is the emotional foundation of each tale that creates the special bond among one's peers.

The narrator is Mary. At the time of the interview, she was 33, had just left a difficult job and was struggling with plans for her future. This was her answer to my question about what got her involved in the system in the first place:

I asked for help—I learned afterwards why it felt so horrible because it was just like someone was reading from a text-book and they weren't listening to me as a person. I had struggled on my own for three years and then I had asked for help and the person promised help and then didn't follow through. It devastated me. I tried to take my life as a result and I ended up in ICU with my family doctor asking, "What happened?" and I said, "I failed." Somehow, I had lost my spirit—the spirit that was fighting to stay alive for three years on my own when I was continually suicidal. I guess the thing was that the power of the system, whether with good intentions or not, tried to destroy the little bit of fight that was left in me. When I said I had failed, I knew I was broken. We're not talking about anything that is outside of me—it's the part that keeps me ticking and it's that part that connects with other consumers and survivors because they know I've been there.

Marg Oswin would support Mary in her views. Marg has a careful, considered way of speaking that belies the passion behind her views. She spoke with me at the offices of an advocacy program where she is a member. Marg is single, in her early fifties and works part-time as an office cleaner for a survivor-run business. She explains further the connection that "having been there" creates.

I entered a convent when I was 18 years old. I left five or six years later because I couldn't find peace within myself, and I wanted to feel differently. Again, looking back, I believe this all stems from the abuse I suffered when I was child. Something was wrong but I didn't know what it was and didn't want to think about it. I began to take drugs. I took valium. I took speed. I took anything that would make me feel different. In 1980, I guess it was, I was taking hands full of valium and wine and things like that and, of course, it led to what the doctors call a psychotic episode and I, well, I was dragged into hospital, kicking and screaming. I withdrew from valium cold turkey. I also got diagnosed and misdiagnosed. I got brain-damaged from ECT. I got lots of different kinds of medication that delayed my taking action against the real problem. So I got 12 or 13 years of postponing work that should have been done a long time ago and that I've been doing now for four years.

> So, I always think of survivors as having a special
> bond. It's unique—maybe I shouldn't say special.
> Because . . . again I'm just working this out as I go . . .
> because the situation that we find ourselves in is that we
> are treated with electroshock and with drugs, things that
> work on the mind. They make us question ourselves and
> our power and reduce us . . . well, I'll speak from my own
> experience, reduced me to being unsure of my ground. I
> became a cipher. And it was only through the support of
> other survivors, and some service providers as well, that I
> was able to pull myself together and find out that I have
> strength and power of my own. With survivors . . . among
> ourselves particularly . . . because we've faced this kind of
> oppression . . . of the mind and of the spirit—and we've all
> experienced it—it's the sharing of a special kind of empti-
> ness and aloneness and despair—and hope—that I haven't
> seen with other forms of oppression.

While most respondents were adamant that they shared
the type of bond that Marg describes, there is a small nuance
that merits mention. Respondents who had *not* experienced
admission as an inpatient to a psychiatric facility tended to
refer to their fellow consumers and survivors as "them" and
"they," while those with inpatient histories more typically
spoke of "we" and "us." While this is admittedly a small point,
it adds depth to the idea that some people experience inpatient
psychiatric treatment as traumatizing and, therefore, as particularly capable of creating a bond among their peers that has
special cohesion.

As a final point, Cassin (1993), herself a psychiatric survivor, believes that the bond which consumers and survivors
presently share is based solely on a mutually acknowledged set
of grievances. While she agrees that consumers' and survivors'
complaints are many, she warns that "grievances [can] become
ends in themselves, rather than problems which must be
solved" (p. 176). The danger lies in creating an esprit de corps
based on a never-ending search for more and more complaints,
siphoning off much-needed energy which should more properly
be focused on creating positive change. She goes on to say that
movements based exclusively on grievances can find themselves
unable to celebrate gains because resolved complaints, instead

of signaling success, represent the frightening erosion of solidarity.

The personal becomes political

The stories respondents told are already indicative of a collectively developed truth because one of the most important audiences for their telling has been each other. In contrast, the few historical examples of patient and ex-patient stories that have survived were told in isolation: to diaries, to unresponsive doctors and, in rare circumstances, to a curious public intrigued by glimpses of life in a madhouse. Nevertheless, these long-ago stories are remarkably similar in content and theme to their contemporary counterparts. Chamberlin (1978), who has listened to literally hundreds of her fellow ex-patients describe their hospital experiences, states that "it's amazing how the same themes, often the same words, occur again and again. . . . [Ex-patients say,] 'You tell them what they want to hear. You learn to play the game'" (p. 68). However, the reality is that these isolated voices have had little overall effect. As one respondent said, "It really frightens me because there isn't even anybody saying this is wrong except one group—the victims of it—and nobody is listening to them."

Chamberlin (1978) believes that, if mental patients want real help, they are going to have to provide it themselves because both psychiatry and professionally developed alternatives have failed. The so-called therapeutic community simply disguised the power of the professional staff who, without a doubt, retained veto power and only permitted patient decisions if they agreed. R.D. Laing never treated his patients as equals, as he claimed, and only believed what they had to say after he translated their words into his own ideas and concepts. The spread of community mental health programs is especially frightening. "Where once the state found it more convenient to incarcerate us permanently, it now seeks to control us through a network of facilities" (Chamberlin, 1978, p. xii). And finally, feminists are seen as especially traitorous because, as women and as fellow oppressed peoples, they ought to know better. Pat Capponi, in a 1992 presentation in Toronto to a group of feminist mental health service providers, advised that there are two classes of women—the workers and the worked-on—and, in many cases, the workers just don't get it. Women who live in violence and poverty have no time for feminist navel-gazing. Keeping themselves fed and their kids out of the Children's Aid is more than a full-time job—with no guarantees of success. Lectures on the hazards of domestic violence have little meaning when the choice is between life on the streets and a roof over your head. In fact, mental health workers' well-intentioned but thoughtless interference can place women in even more danger. In comparison, professionals go home at night, in cars, to a safe neighbourhood and a family. Who are you, Capponi asks, to define our needs, and why do you think you can give advice when you have so little understanding of the true nature of our lives? As for feminist therapy, "how does an hour of talk change the fact that incest, rape, battery and harassment are cultural norms?" (Raymond et al., 1982). Capponi's view of therapy is equally clear. Nobody, she says, is going to mess with her head.

In 1971, the Vancouver Mental Patients Association began operation as the first organization completely run by and for "users" of the mental health system. In the United States, the self-help movement was delayed somewhat because of a less welcoming funding climate, but today Chamberlin (1990) describes the rise of mutual aid among American consumers and psychiatric survivors as a strikingly successful phenomenon. Ironically, despite a promising beginning, self-help in Canada has had a lesser impact. Hardie (as quoted in Everett, 1994a) states that the reason for this disparity is one of the downsides of the Canadian social welfare and health care system. In Canada, the establishment of self-help can be seen as biting the hand that feeds as well as competing with professional interests. As a consequence, many self-help initiatives have suffered from a strong professional presence, often negating their very purpose (Everett & Shimrat, 1993).

Self-help organizations create a welcoming environment for the incubation of collective mistrust. Personal stories, such as those told by this study's respondents, find a sympathetic audience among peers and have become a hallmark of the "self-help way." Gamson (1991) calls mutual aid organizations "movement halfway houses." Self-help groups serve to create "an environment in which a collective action consciousness is fostered, personal skills are enhanced, knowledge of earlier struggles is acquired and a vision of a future society is developed" (Gamson, 1991, p. 38). Stories, when told to one's fellows, name the "self as a site for politicization" (hooks, 1989, p. 106) and foster feelings of mutuality and community, nested within a burgeoning sense of political purpose. However, by their very nature, these stories emphasize one main aspect of personhood and concentrate principally on one set of experiences. The process of making the personal political adds social dimensions and implications to these sorts of narrowly focused individual stories, but in a particular way. It makes the "distinction between experiencing a form of exploitation and understanding the particular structure of domination that caused it" (hooks, 1989, p. 108). Politicization is the attempt to move beyond merely a shared understanding of grievances so that a connection with the wider social world can be established, but in a way that is aware of its flaws and of how its structure can wound or even annihilate certain groups of people simply because they are outside the universe of obligation (Gamson, 1995). In the micro sense, a political act "recognizes implicitly the existence of another member of the power relationship" (Janeway, 1980, p. 222). Politicized movement members, in this case consumers and psychiatric survivors, have acquired a critical lens, and, in doing so, have come to "see" and "know" themselves as social beings embedded in a web of power relationships (Prilleltensky & Gonick, 1996).

One of the goals of my research was to understand the process by which consumers and survivors connected the personal with the political. Donna, who asked to be identified by her first name only, told her story in response to this question. She is 39 years old, married with one son.

Donna's father died when she was a baby and, in retrospect, she thinks that her mother slipped into a deep depression and never really got over it. Eventually, Donna herself became depressed. "Maybe I just learned how to be depressed or maybe my emotional needs weren't met because I was being cared for by a depressed person." Whatever the case, Donna began seeing psychiatrists as a teenager and refers to them as "poor man's therapists" because their fees are covered by Medicare. Even though Donna had never been hospitalized on a psychiatric ward, she, too, felt betrayed by the failure of the psychiatric power contract. "I expected that I would be told why I was depressed, how to get over it and how to move on with my life. What I got was nothing. I asked questions and I got no answers." Eventually, Donna got a job as the staff member to the Patient Council[1] in a provincial psychiatric hospital. One of the tasks of the Council is to deal with complaints from patients. It was here that she feels the process of politicization began for her.

> I'll tell you, I had an experience in here. We were dealing with a patient and she had quite a lot of valid concerns and complaints so I just went through the normal routine to get them addressed. The things that happened to her . . . I mean, she was beaten up. She used to go home and visit her son on weekends and after her complaint, the very first weekend she came back, she had a bag of things with her and they did a search and seizure which they do if they feel you're a threat. She'd been checking out of this ward for a year on weekends and they never searched her once and this day, they searched her stuff and beat her up because she resisted. It was just incredible.
>
> And her psychologist would bring her to tears by reminding her that she was suicidal. I mean, the things that happened to her were so atrocious, but many were so subtle that you couldn't make a complaint that was concrete. It was all innuendo and it was insidious what they did. They really tried to destroy this girl because she made a few complaints.
>
> So we talked to her endlessly about dependency on the system, about what the health care providers have to offer and, I mean, this was not our political tirade. It was

---

1 Patient Councils were created in Ontario's provincial psychiatric hospitals as yet another expression of consumer and psychiatric survivor participation. Money was allocated to hire consumer and survivor staff to facilitate the recruitment of a group composed of, usually, outpatients who acted as advisors to administration. Councils have also developed for themselves a kind of watchdog role, offering a place where inpatients can take complaints.

her coming to the realization that they couldn't help her. And they switched her wards and then the talk around the hospital was that they were all waiting for her to attempt suicide so that the Patient Council could get blamed for it. It was just an awful experience.

Finally, this young lady left. She signed herself out of the hospital. We've kept in touch with her. It's been a year and a half now and she's doing very well. I mean, she's not working but she's certainly looking after her son and her husband and she's functioning and doing some advocacy work for people in the community. She has bad days just like everybody does, but the point is that if she had believed what they said, I think she would be dead. And she chose to decide that they were not going to help her. She had to struggle through whatever this was herself, with her own methods and her own means. And she did. And she came out on top. I look at her now as a particularly strong individual but if you had seen her at the time, I mean, they had her in tears all the time and she was always upset. And she was always in trouble.

And I'm not blaming it on the health care professionals. I'm simply saying that they're part of this social construct and they're the reinforcing tool. Once you get here, man, they plant these ideas in you for sure. So, for me, watching this little girl who just made a small complaint at the beginning . . . well, I know now you cannot win. You cannot win, no matter what you do. Except to follow the rules. The more you do what you're told, the more likely you are to get out. You don't get better. You don't learn how to stand up for yourself. You just get out.

While Donna couldn't be clearer about the triggers that led to her politicization, Susan Marshall says that her route was a "long, complicated process."

At first, I hid. Then, I did the "I'm the only one this has happened to" route—which, of course, meant that I couldn't do anything about it. As I discovered my peers and I discovered that I wasn't the only one this has happened to . . . the more I heard, the angrier I got, that's for sure. So it was sort of the process—along with deciding what to do about it . . . deciding actually what was wrong about it or what was *in common* wrong with it.

Sometimes, as Mary explains, it's just one thing, an experience that sheds light where none existed before. The psychiatric facility in which Mary was a patient is one of the few in Canada that is funded through both private and public means. As a result, the patients, too, are divided—some are public and others are private. She says:

> We are all supposed to be equal. The public beds are supposed to be for those who are most in need, but the people are treated *very* differently than those in the private beds. So I signed myself out. My doctor said, "Mary, you cannot separate the politics from your own healing." And the last day I was there I said, "That's unrealistic." The reality is that that's part of me. My healing is personal, but the politics, I just can't help but see the politics.

Jennifer Chambers would agree with Mary. Jennifer, like Donna, is employed as staff to the Patient Council at the former Queen Street Mental Health Centre. She originally trained as a psychologist, completing part of her master's degree. We met for a drink in a bar near my office and the background noise nearly drowned out her quiet voice. I have occasionally witnessed Jennifer in action in her public role as a psychiatric survivor advocate, and I have come to the conclusion that the gentleness of her voice is an effective tool for capturing the attention of her listeners so that she can deliver her razor-sharp critiques. At 37, Jennifer is a step-parent, which she says is "a very formal way of describing my relationship to the two teenagers I live with." She also wants it known that her identity as a psychiatric survivor is not her *whole* life.

When Jennifer was a teenager, she attempted suicide after "giving out fairly noisy signals that fell on deaf ears." She was subsequently hospitalized, and, when she tried to leave, was committed on an involuntary basis. In order to get out, she appeared before a group of professionals, in the company of her mother, to prove that she was sane—which, she says, "I'd defy anyone to do." She had hoped that the hospital staff would "help her get what was inside out." However, not long after she was admitted, a ward social worker told her that if she didn't "snap out of it," she would be given electro-convulsive therapy.

"I learned quickly to pretend that I was fine which, of course, was the problem in the first place."

However, it's not solely Jennifer's hospitalization experience that led to her political beliefs. Instead, she credits her present job and her brief experience as a professional with "opening her eyes."

> It's hard to separate my politics from my feelings. I used to have a position that was sort of more empathetic to all sides and I'd say that the work I've done in the last few years has made me angrier . . . battering my head up against the brick wall of the Ministry of Health and the hospital administration. It's harder to see the humanity of the people I'm dealing with than it used to be because I'm not treated with humanity. In a way, I think it was a relief for me to discover the psychiatric survivor perspective because when I was working as a professional counsellor, there was a discomfort with the sense that I was always kind of putting something over on the other person. It's partly because I had experienced the other side so I'm more sensitive to it. It's very difficult to be natural in either role and they *are* roles. When I started the co-counselling that I do, I found a philosophy that was compatible with my own so that gave me an initial sense of support for my views and eventually the survivor movement provided the political analysis which I think is a power analysis. It was somehow a relief to be able to share with people my experience of being hospitalized, to say, "OK, I'm one of you." I think that if I hadn't started peer counselling, I might have tried to forget my hospital experience but I'd have kept the shame.

Three other respondents spoke of their politicization in this way:

Adele Rosenbloom:

> I was a political woman. I was a feminist. I was involved in a lot of anti-war activities. I had that framework but I didn't have the psychiatric survivor framework. That came after meeting other people who had similar experiences and hearing their stories and hearing about the oppression. It made me very angry and I had this great need to speak out and organize and go to demos and try to change things.

Walter Osoka:

> I think when something is done to you in a very conde-
> scending, very deleterious way—where you lose your place
> of residence, where you lose your self-respect, where you
> lose a significant other . . . where your whole being drops
> to such a level. . . . You can either fight or you can drown. I
> chose to fight and . . . and it, well, it leaves a person want-
> ing to help. Which doesn't mean you come out swinging at
> everything you see. It just means that you have a healthy
> cynicism, a healthy need to get involved, to take your
> lumps. You also have a healthy respect for people in your
> own situation and a desire to go and look for the people
> who somehow figure that simply because they have all
> these degrees, they should be listened to more than other
> people who haven't. And say to them, "Get off Mount
> Olympus and get down here."

Patrick Brown:

> Well, I don't consider myself an activist. No, I don't. I just
> think that I do what needs to be done. Speak up when
> somebody needs to speak up. There's a saying that goes
> like this: "When good men sit back and do nothing, evil
> triumphs." And I'm a full believer . . . a *total* believer in
> that because I feel that if I can contribute to the system, to
> society, then a lot of injustices will be corrected, so that's
> why I do what I do.

These comments and the ones that precede them confirm
and expand upon Lord and Hutchison's (1993) findings on the
process of personal empowerment. Indeed, people must first
get angry, but beyond this there are at least two paths to politicization for consumers and survivors. First, they may base their
new way of seeing the world on their own experiences, which
take on greater significance when shared with peers. Alternatively, they may witness others' experiences and, through these
vicarious means, come to embrace a politicized identity. Either
way, their new-found mistrust and doubt require the validation
of community. "Few people have the strength to stand up for
what they believe in the face of almost unanimous opposition"
(Chamberlin, 1978, p. 75). There is an extraordinary pressure on
consumers and survivors to see their problems as exclusively of

their own making. The express purpose of psychiatric diagnosis is the appropriation of individual experience in preparation for translation into medicalized terminology, thereby fulfilling the twin goals of localizing the problem as within the "diseased" person and capturing it for professional intervention. But it is a suspicious circumstance when biology appears to be a destiny only for the powerless (Janeway, 1980). By coming together to share stories and create bonds, consumers and psychiatric survivors have discovered what Susan Marshall did—that their experiences have something *in common*. Once the discovery is made, one form of protest would be a reprise of the resistance strategy that got them out of the psychiatric hospital in the first place. They could turn their backs on the whole thing and leave. However, the respondents in this study have chosen to stay, in large measure because they have access to a previously unavailable avenue for expressing dissatisfaction—political activism and non-violent protest in the form of the consumer and psychiatric survivor movement. Indeed, respondents affirm, in colloquial terms, that their experiences have left them "fighting mad." As some feminist survivors have said:

> Our anger is real. Our anger at our experiences of oppression as women and as psychiatric inmates, of being raped, beaten, locked up, drugged, shocked, is valid and strong. It is not a "symptom" to be drugged or therapized away. It is, instead, our source of power, a fuel for our outrage and our activism. (Raymond et al., 1982, p. 8)

In conclusion

De Certeau (1984) states that "the acceptance of a limitation is the foundation of a social contract" (p. 64). Donna puts it more clearly. She says people tend to think that "if you asked for help, you should put up with whatever you get." Asking for help carries with it an implicit agreement between the powerful and the powerless that the right to protest, complain or perhaps even comment on what's offered is forfeit. However, fundamental changes in social power structures that relate to new, more egalitarian ways of distributing knowledge have created an opening for do-it-yourself alternatives to the psychiatric system. After a process of recapturing their own identities, consumers and psychiatric survivors have had the previously denied option of sharing their stories among one another. As a result, they have awakened a collective sense of anger in response to what they view as the trauma of many forms of psychiatric help. However, as these stories demonstrate, respondents appear unable to identify these sorts of changes as powerful expressions of agency which are capable, at least potentially, of great impact. In addition, Cassin (1993) warns that a movement founded solely on grievances has a limited future because it can only survive by finding more and more complaints to sustain itself. Nevertheless, consumers' and survivors' increased visibility and often critical presence at many levels of the Ontario mental health system, recent though it may be, has definitely had an impact. One of the more interesting effects has been their stance towards mental health professionals. Given that for literally centuries psychiatrists and other professionals have defined who consumers and survivors are, it is indeed interesting to see how consumers and survivors, in their long awaited turn, define who mental health professionals are.

6

Them

The evolution of an identity that is independent of the one that has been developed by the dominant forces "creates boundaries between an 'us' and a 'them'" (Gamson, 1991, p. 42). From a philosophical perspective, there must be an "I" in order for there to be a "you." In other words, a subject requires an object and, in de Beauvoir's (1949) pioneering feminist example, women are the objects of men's subjectivity— they are Other. The primary characteristic of the category of Other is that its members have no substance of their own and, thus, they have only a secondary role to play in the project of life. They are not, however, useless because they are the mirrors in which dominant subjects search for their own reflections. Subjects and objects have a relationship which in Janeway's (1980) language is called a power contract.

The psychiatric gaze has historically rested upon a group of people who now call themselves consumers and psychiatric survivors and who, in the last few decades, have begun to gaze back. The struggle to reappropriate their own "spoiled identity" (Goffman, 1963) and celebrate it individually and collectively has meant the development of a group history. It includes a set of "mythologies" which defines a site for the launching of an embryonic subjectivity, complete with a clear picture of its own version of Other. The consumer and psychiatric survivor category of Other is composed of psychiatrists and other mental health professionals.

This chapter represents one of the surprises that are so often a part of research. I was well aware of what "we," as professionals, thought of "them," the patients, at least from the perspective of my own experience as a staff person in a psychiatric hospital, but I didn't anticipate the pivotal role that professionals play in consumers' and survivors' internal and external life worlds, although de Beauvoir certainly would have. She states, "Once the subject seeks to assert himself, the Other, who limits and denies him, is none the less a necessity to him: he attains himself only through that reality which he is not" (1949, p. 157). Psychiatric survivor Chrystine Cassin (1993) adds, "*We* create an image of *them*: we look in our mirror and affirm that we are not like *them. They* do the same thing with respect to *us*. When we begin to refuse to allow them to re-mold, re-create us into their image of what we ought to be, then the battle lines are drawn" (p. 375).

Invisibility

People who reside within the universe of obligation may not be transgressed against without consequences. However, actions against outsiders are often ignored or may even be legally sanctioned (Gamson, 1995). Exclusion from the universe of obligation requires a visibility which is accorded the group but, paradoxically, denied the individual.

In consumers' and survivors' lives, there appear to be four aspects to invisibility. First, there is the type of invisibility that can serve as a protective measure employed to evade the scrutiny of the powerful. This sort of invisibility offers only relative safety and the cost is silence (Gamson, 1995). In the previous chapter, Donna described what happens when a patient shed her invisibility in order to complain about her hospital treatment.

Consumers and psychiatric survivors report that complaining, when not in an institution, more typically invokes the second aspect of invisibility—being discounted. Esso Leete describes it this way: "I can talk, but I may not be heard. I can make suggestions, but they may not be taken seriously. I can voice my thoughts, but they may be seen as delusions. I can recite experiences, but they may be interpreted as fantasies" (as quoted in Deegan, 1990). Bonnie Burstow (1992) offers a concrete example of what can happen when patients are discounted. In the early 1970s, a woman patient of James Tyhurst, the psychiatrist who lent his name to the famed Ontario mental health policy document *More for the Mind* (Tyhurst et al., 1963), complained of blatant and cruel sexual abuse involving master-slave scenarios, forced fellatio and whippings. Tyhurst was not charged until approximately 14 years later when three more former patients came forward with the same or similar stories. Tyhurst's defense was that his patients were delusional and, therefore, could not be believed. He was only convicted because experts agreed that the complainants' diagnoses, borderline personality disorder, did not involve delusions, adding that, had they been schizophrenic, Tyhurst may very likely have been set free (Burstow, in *OPSAnews #1*, 1990). As a second illustration of this type of invisibility, one of the present study's respondents offers her views on the experience of being discounted:

> Well, ultimately there's that "thing." I had someone say it to me explicitly. I was doing some Board development work at an organization and a woman looked me right in the face and said, "You're mentally ill. How do you know what's good for you?" And I think that pretty much sums it up. It just doesn't matter what you say because everything is pathologized. I tell someone to fuck off, I have an anger management problem. A normal person tells someone to fuck off, they're just angry. You know what I mean? Everything we do is pathologized. I do this work (at a drop-in centre), and the shrinks tell me, "You do that work to avoid facing your own issues." So, I don't do this work, then I'm avoiding responsibility. Once you get the label, you just might as well accept that everything that comes out of your mouth is not going to be legitimated, so I'm working on the premise that nobody takes me seriously and I try to go from there.

Consumers and survivors also report that they experience invisibility when they seek help from the mental health system. The following speaker is Sue Goodwin who, at 32, sometimes wonders why she is still alive.

> I threw myself in front of a subway when I was 23 because I
> was still going through all the flashbacks and memories of
> sexual abuse and thinking nobody loved me and there I was,
> a successful woman with a job and a husband and going
> places in my career and I jumped in front of a subway at
> lunch time. Because I still had the thought from childhood
> that nobody loved me, you know? The system didn't help me
> because I had been going to see a psychiatrist while I was at
> work and I was on masses of medication to zip me up in the
> morning and to calm me down at night so that I could func-
> tion at work, as a wife and as a social being with friends.
> And it just didn't work. All that so-called intervention didn't
> help a bit because nobody talked to me and nobody listened.

The final aspect of invisibility is experienced as a result of
interactions with "them" in consumers' and survivors' political
roles. Cassin (1993) calls it the "vanishing principle" (p. 374),
and Jennifer Chambers offers an example:

> The first time I was at an event that included mental health
> professionals and I was there identifying as a survivor was a
> conference that we had about four years ago. It was amazing
> to me because I had been studying in the mental health
> system as a student and I'd worked in the system as a re-
> searcher—and my experience when people knew I was a sur-
> vivor was so different. I was so ignored! I was in a session
> looking at, what was it now? I think it was education or
> something. The session was chaired by a psychiatrist and
> one of the things I was trying to suggest was that the lan-
> guage should be changed so that when they talk about
> expertise and education, instead, talk about knowledge and
> experience which would include first-hand knowledge. And
> although he wrote down everything that everyone else said,
> when I spoke, he wouldn't write it down. Other people in the
> room started to notice. I was even saying, "You could write
> that down . . . right there . . . under that category." And it
> didn't matter. It was as if I wasn't speaking. It was eerie.

They hate emotion

Respondents reported that the one thing guaranteed
to make mental health professionals uncomfortable is a display
of emotion. Walter Osoka lives in London. At the time I spoke

with him, he was studying at Fanshaw College, hoping to get work in the social services. He says, "I show emotion which people hate, especially service providers. Why is that?" Jennifer Chambers diagnoses the problem this way:

> People have to be prepared to go through some pain in order to move forward, and something the mental health system teaches people is NEVER to allow that to happen. If you feel pain, immediately suppress it with drugs.

Indeed, in recent decades, critics of psychiatry argue that by emphasizing biological factors in the etiology of mental illness, the profession has turned increasingly to pharmacological solutions and electro-convulsive therapy to the neglect of the wider social and psychological contexts of patients' lives (Breggin, 1991). Childhood trauma, disturbing life events, violence, poverty, loss and grief are seen as affecting the course of illness (Goff et al., 1991), but are relegated to marginal status in psychiatric treatment plans (Beiser, 1990; Joffe et al., 1989). These concerns may figure more prominently in the paradigms of the other mental health disciplines, but this sort of compartmentalization of life experience leaves people like Mary feeling "divided up." She says:

> Professionals offer a kind of segmented helping. They say, "I can only give you this much. You now have to go to the social worker for that, or the nurse for the other thing" and each may call themselves "person-centred," but I am fragmented and my whole person is not dealt with. They're always saying, "That's social worky kind of stuff so we can't do that together. I do therapy kind of stuff." So I'm left running around in circles because I just don't know where the answer is.

Mary's experiences are perhaps indicative of the fragmentation in the professional mind. Indeed, now as in the past, the professional view on the role of environment versus biology in the etiology of mental illness is "divided up," often expressed as a duel between conflicting sets of research findings. Reminiscent of R.D. Laing, Peter Breggin (1991), a contemporary antipsychiatry proponent, calls mental illness "psychospiritual overwhelm," and places a strong emphasis on the need for professionals to understand patients' emotional lives. To shore up his argument, he meticulously documents the flaws and misconceptions that he feels pass for bona fide psychiatric research findings. In addition, Illich (1975) argues that the paramount goal of the medical enterprise has been to "detach pain from any subjective or inter-subjective context in order to annihilate it" (p. 93). In doing so, it has also usurped control, separating the individual sufferer from the responsibility inherent in the management of his or her own pain. Illich believes that pain, in all its forms, is a challenge to human beings which calls them to attention and forces interpretation. It poses a question that cries out for an answer. It makes people think as well as feel. Sometimes it must be endured and, at other times, conquered, but it always requires a response even if that response can only be courage.

Donna would concur. She states:

> You have to learn that your pain is part of you. I'm not saying you should cheer about the atrocities that have happened to you, but they're part of what makes you the person you are. I think you have to learn to deal with that stuff, to live with it, to accept it and move on. We know there's not a lot of evidence that cognitive therapy does anything. I really believe that all therapy is is picking scabs to watch them bleed. Clients never get better and therapists are just picking, picking, picking. People always feel crappy in therapy. So, I think you have to learn that it's OK to be where you are, that you don't have a disease, that you're not different from other people, and that you have value.

However, many respondents report that they were unable to "accept it and move on," as Donna advises. "If I'd known how to make myself feel better, I would have done so long ago," says Jane Pritchard, a 20-year veteran of multiple admissions to psychiatric hospitals. Jane is a former librarian who maintained her employment between her inpatient stays and has only recently retired. She speaks of the pain in her life before she entered the "system":

The only way I had of coping with my life was to be seriously depressed. I lived with that for many years and finally, one day, I said, "I can't live like this one moment longer. I thought I had to kill myself because I didn't know there was any way of helping me to be anything other than depressed. However, that was such an incredibly . . . such a serious decision, I thought about it and I said to myself, "Well Jane, once you do it, you don't get to change your mind. Surely, there must be someone out there that you can go to for help." I figured I needed help from the experts. However, that's not what I got. I got abuse. All kinds of abuse.

Mary describes a similar experience this way:

Most of my energy was going into just surviving and I wasn't able to contribute to my community, to society in the way that I knew I could. So it was a constant struggle and it just got worse and worse. I mean, I was trying, but I didn't think I could do it myself. I thought that I must need to know something else, something outside of me. . . . My whole life just seemed out of control. . . . So in 1989, I reached out for help, hoping that the professionals would listen and actually work with me but that's not what I got. It didn't matter what I felt. What got lost was my personhood.

Walter concludes that professionals hate emotional pain because that's "the way they've been educated." He goes on to point out how men's pain may not, in fact, be ignored. Instead, it is misinterpreted.

Have you ever heard this? What's the flip side of depression? Professionals call it anger. If you're depressed . . . especially if you're a guy, what you really are is angry. This is what I was told. I'm not making it up! See, if I have any type of emotion, if I cry it's because I'm angry. If I laugh hysterically, I'm angry. If I hug somebody, which I don't do very well, but if I show any kind of emotion, it's because I'm angry. If I was to give a speech, if I show emotion, if I break down and I cry or whatever because I'm so emotional about a certain thing, it's not because it's something that was very dear to me, it's because I'm angry.

Church (1993) agrees with Walter when he says that mental health professionals are educated in such a way as to suppress their own and others' emotional lives. She believes that professionals feel required to conform to a certain behavioural code which she describes as: "Don't give offense. Don't be unpleasant or adversarial. Don't complain or fight. Be nice. Be reasonable. Be considerate. Be cooperative" (p. 210). Church concludes that professionals trade in their ability to express emotion, especially anger, in return for membership in the inner circle of power—the universe of obligation. On the other hand, psychiatric survivors, in both their patient and political roles, are not constrained in the same way. She quotes one survivor as saying: "Most of the unwritten rules affect the mental health professionals rather than us survivors. . . . We don't have jobs that are at the mercy of anyone. . . . We have nothing to lose, absolutely nothing to lose and everything to gain" (p. 218). While it must be noted that these comments were made prior to the advent of the Consumer/Survivor Development Initiative, which today employs many consumers and survivors in jobs they would be loath to lose, they are nevertheless instructive. Having nothing to lose, while typically the most powerless of social positions, can in some circumstances constitute a powerful advantage. Consumers and survivors need not hold their tongues or quell their emotions in fear of losing status. In addition, having at one time or another acquired the label "crazy," they can, if they so chose, exploit with relative impunity the political potential of this stigmatized identity, locating themselves outside the reach of many of the social niceties, courtesies and polite interactional rules that professionals must follow. In fact, the occasional "bad manners" of loud, emotional confrontation give consumers and survivors a powerful edge (Church, 1996).

It's just a job

Albrecht (1992) states that life's problems are expressed in sets of social relationships which, by themselves, have no formally acknowledged meaning. Meaning is attributed only when responsibility, language, symbols and values are assigned. If a problem is given a psychiatric meaning, then solutions are to be provided by the mental health system. In other words, it is a system that depends on the appropriation of life problems for its existence and, while it is the individual that feels the distress, it is the system that defines the need. And these needs are great and ever increasing. "The health care industry . . . is one of the largest clusters of economic activity in all modern states" (Evans & Stoddart, 1994, p. 27). By extension, it is also one of the largest employers of professional helpers.

Chamberlin (1978) believes that there is a fundamental difference between help which is offered altruistically, from one human being to another, and help that has been professionalized. When helpers are financially rewarded for caring, it is natural and perhaps even necessary to suspect a conflict of motives. The end result of the formal, paid mental health system is that it creates and perpetuates a chasm between the well, normal helper and the sick, abnormal patient. Chamberlin states, "detachment and impartiality, which mental health professionals believe are the proper therapeutic attitudes, become, in practice, either cold formality or the shallow pretense of friendliness" (p. 149). Asking for help, she concludes, will never be shorn of its inherent humiliation until our culture recognizes that all people need help and support at some time in their lives and, when they do, it is normal to ask for it.

Patrick Brown was born in Jamaica but has lived in Canada since he was a teenager. When he first entered the system, he felt that it would take a month or two to get back on his feet. "But to my surprise, it took me 15 years to get to that place. I don't think that anybody could have snapped their fingers and got me well. I think it was a process." At 38, Patrick now works at a job opportunity project for consumers and survivors. He says he has met a lot of good people in the system but the person who helped him the most wasn't a psychiatrist or a professional. It was a friend.

> I think the people who are the most effective are those who are compassionate. We need more empathy and you can't pay somebody to be empathetic—you can't pay somebody to care. It has to come from the heart. I mean, if you are making $50 an hour working as a therapist and they decide

to give you $200 an hour, you might do something differently but I don't think it would make you a more empathetic person. Money changes people, but I don't think money can change things like that.

Hugh Tapping argues that the advocacy efforts of mental health professionals are also suspect because they have competing interests—what they say they want on behalf of "us patients" is closely tied to the things that promote the status of their own profession. Hugh is a survivor of the "good old, bad old days," spending his seventeenth birthday in a psychiatric institution receiving numerous rounds of ECT. He is also a veteran of the mental patient liberation movement of the early seventies. At 46, he says that the best way to describe him is to say that "words and wit are not necessarily the same as wisdom." He offers his view on how professionals promote their own self-interest.

> For example, when professionals began to talk about the "mentally ill" rather than the insane, this was just an earlier version of what is, today, called politically correct language. The public doesn't care about these kinds of terms—they're mostly irrelevant to them. The idea of being "mentally ill" didn't come from us. It was another one of these top-down things done by professionals who are in a position of privilege and power. Its biggest result was that it reduced a lot of the stigma of working with us crazy people. It used to be that you work in the loony bin, people look at you funny just like they look at us patients and now, well, gosh, you must be a nice, helpful, professional. And, of course, this was also correlated with a rather significant across-the-board increase in income levels for those non-medical doctors we call psychiatrists.

Donna says:

> There is no one fighting for the rights of the mentally ill unless you count the caregivers and then that's a completely different story. What we're talking about is a growth industry in a time of diminishing career paths. So, they say people are best stabilized in a community-based crisis program and it's clear that their next job will be in a community-based crisis program, well . . . I'm not saying

this to be cynical. I don't think professionals are in this with malicious intent, but you have to, at all times, question their motives. They're coming from a skewed vantage point.

Jennifer Chambers gives an example of this "skewed vantage point":

> The power of the written word is not overlooked by the powers-that-be. For example, our article in *The Toronto Star* about rights violations at the hospital—the next day the associate administrator had been by our office about five times and wanted to meet about it and he said he was very upset about this article and we said, "Why don't you get upset about the rights violations instead of being upset about seeing it in print?"

These respondents seem in agreement with the oft-repeated consumer and psychiatric survivor charge that the mental health system profits from their misery. Patrick argues that human compassion is not for sale. Others add that, when push comes to shove and jobs or reputations are at stake, the professionals' economic well-being will come first. But, as Jane Pritchard says, "if they would just do their jobs, do what they are paid for—listen to us, treat us like human beings with brains and emotions, and provide real help," then the integrity of the power contract would be preserved.

They are abusive

True to their historical tradition, consumers and psychiatric survivors seek to expose abuse in the mental health system. Contemporary activists make the distinction between two levels of abuse. First, there is what they would call sanctioned abuse, psychiatric treatment itself. Second, there is abuse that would be called criminal by anyone's standards.

In a 1989 broadcast on the CBC, Irit Shimrat, aided by many of her peers, talked about the types of abuse—as they define it—that pass for psychiatric "help."

> Last year, I was picked up by the cops. I'm a small person. I weigh 118 pounds. They tied me in four-point restraint to a stretcher in Mount Sinai Hospital here in Toronto. I kept

> getting out of the restraints and eventually I was put in a leather harness and that's when I was injected with Haldol. I was paralyzed from the waist down. I couldn't talk. My jaw was completely locked. (p. 2)

> The medication was so heavy, none of the patients knew what was going on. And when my children came to visit me at the Royal Ottawa, they wept because Mummy was so out of it. (p. 5)

> I calculated I had at least 50 or 60 insulin shocks. It succeeded in making me scared as hell and I shut up—it worked by inducing fear. (p. 4)

> They ripped my clothes off and stuck me in the bum with needles very painfully and roughly because I was struggling to get away from them. (p. 11)

> I was rendered instantly unconscious. My body, a few seconds later, entered into convulsive seizures. A lethal electrocution consists of one ampere for one second through your brain. What we're talking about is more than half of a lethal electrocution, each and every time. This is called therapy. (p. 19)

Many respondents had their own stories of abuse to tell, some of which are reported in the preceding chapter. Hugh Tapping adds:

> It's all very well to acknowledge that many people come from abusive families, but who's going to acknowledge that abuse goes on in institutions and by professionals. Are we going to acknowledge that when you're in a disproportionate power relationship, disproportionate things happen? Whether you're a kid or an adult, when you're driven crazy by an abusive situation in your family, you are likely to be forced into an abusive situation in an institution. And if you get your act a bit more together and you go looking for an "alternative" therapist—although I've got a lot of respect for what a lot of people do—I don't see any more quality assurance mechanisms in place in a community agency than I see in the run-of-the-mill big, bad institution.

The second type of abuse is that which is defined by the Roeher Institute Report (Roeher Institute, 1995). It highlights the extreme vulnerability of people who are dependent on their caregivers. In the context of this study, a respondent described one such experience as follows:

> I flipped out once and my landlady called the police. I was self-injuring. I have a history of self-inflicted violence. And that was the one time the police took me to a hospital, but there were no beds so they took me to this other "safe" place and one of the other people staying there raped me. So I thought, well, this is fucking crazy, right? Like, this system is fucked. On the streets, I know how to take care of myself. Locked in this place, I can't take care of myself.

Some respondents, however, felt that professionals don't intend to be unkind and abusive. They just don't get it. Walter Osoka says:

> The whole idea of professionalism is fine except that they are stuck at doing a certain thing a certain way and some-times they don't look at the broader picture. It's kind of like, "Take a Prozac and call me in two weeks." But I'm hungry. I have no place to stay. I have no friends. I have no communication with other people. "Well, that's OK. This will make you fine anyway."

Patrick Brown also believes that they really don't mean it:

> A lot of injustices are done in the name of psychiatry but I don't think those injustices are purposely done. I don't think the psychiatrists or the professionals or the social workers or whatever set out to be unjust. It's something that happened by chance or happened because they didn't take the time to listen. They didn't take the time to analyze the situation.

Donna concurs:

> What I realized was that the caregivers are not hurting us intentionally. They buy into this. They believe that they have the answers . . . that they have the education, that they've read exactly the right number of books they need to tell somebody what's wrong with them and to fix them. They *believe* that. What they don't realize is that people are dying because of it.

Janeway (1980) is not as lenient in her views of the motivations of the powerful. She states that what they want to do is remake the minds of their subjects, but "the mind can only be remade in one way, by recapitulating the process of socialization through which individuals learned the world and came to maturity" (p. 207). Certainly, Hugh Tapping refers to what he sees as the interconnectivity of abuse in families, institutions and, possibly, community mental health services. People fleeing abusive families, he says, find themselves in abusive psychiatric hospitals and, upon discharge, in abusive boarding homes and, potentially, in abusive community-based programs. Other respondents also alluded to the frustration they feel when they ask for help and find that the factors that precipitated their distress in the first place are recapitulated in the "help" they are offered. Miller (1983), in speaking of professional education, says that it's no wonder that people who themselves have spent years in repressive institutions of higher learning victimize their patients and clients. "Students . . . are spending four years at the universities learning to regard human beings as machines in order to gain a better understanding of how they function . . . [instead of] unmasking the devastating consequences of the way power is secretly exercised under the guise of child-rearing" (p. 278). She concludes that because children are punished for awareness and understanding, as adults they give up the quest, preferring the false safety of ignorance while, in shame, repeating the same acts of violation of which they themselves were once victims.

Viewed through the eyes of consumers and survivors, mental health professionals, in general, are not an attractive group of people. They espouse a narrow and inaccurate "caregiving" paradigm, which discounts the views of the people they are supposed to be caring for. They are cut off from their own emotional lives. They are either unthinkingly or maliciously abusive. They look out for number one and, if threatened, quickly drop what appears to be only a thin veneer of high-minded altruism in favour of the cold, hard cash of a paycheque. They develop institutions, programs, theories and treatments that recreate and extend the very problems they are supposed to ameliorate. In short, "they" seem to provide an excellent background against which consumers and survivors can create the foreground of their new identities—"we" must aspire to be everything "they" are not.

But they're more like us than they think

As respondents looked into the mirror provided by their observations of mental health professionals, they noted that what they often saw was themselves. Marilyn Nearing says:

> We had a week-long workshop with consumers and mental health professionals in attendance and I heard them saying the very same things as us. "I'm not in control. There's no money . . . no support." There were front-line staff who clearly didn't know what their agency budgets were. They weren't taking personal responsibility, just like consumers don't take responsibility over their own medications and their own therapy. I saw that commonality between the two. The same sounds of hopelessness. The same sounds of dependency. It rather frightened me because if the front-line staff aren't empowered, how can they pass the power along to their clients?

Jennifer Chambers offers her observations:

> A woman counsellor that I knew gave a talk at Queen Street on sexual abuse and ritual abuse, saying that what is often seen to be psychosis can be flashbacks, and to the staff she said, "Abuse is widespread. Some of you have been abused. If you haven't dealt with that, you're not going to be able to help anyone else." Well, most of the staff walked out. The *insistence* that they are different from the people they serve is so strong.

During her many inpatient stays in a psychiatric hospital, Jane Pritchard says that she often felt alone and suicidal and what she longed for was someone who would "talk to me, listen to me. Help me understand me." She reports that, occasionally late at night when things were quieter, the nurses might sit with her, but the topic of conversation was *their* troubled lives, not hers. These professionals concluded that the kind of help they were offering would never be the kind of help they would seek for their own difficulties.

> I recall one nurse telling me about her sad life and she
> said, "I'm seriously considering committing suicide myself
> but, let me tell you, Jane, I'd never put myself in the posi-
> tion you're in.'

Chamberlin (1978) believes that the enormous distance
between patients and staff in mental institutions makes real
human-to-human interaction impossible. However, revealing
conversations do occur from time to time, indicating that staff
are people who have problems too. But, as Jane's experience
shows, they also recognize that placing themselves in the very
helping hands that they represent is humiliating and shameful
and, as a result, likely to be no help at all. Walter Osoka offers a
variation on this theme. He feels that if mental health professionals themselves understood what it was like to need help and
support, they might be more compassionate. He says, "It's my
hope that people who work in the mental health system will say,
'I've had problems too,' because if they would do that, maybe
getting help wouldn't be such a scary thing." Marilyn Nearing
adds:

> When you look at the really caring and committed profes-
> sionals, you'll probably find out that they've had some sort
> of family or personal experience that has sensitized them. I
> think that when professionals start to admit they belong to
> the same group as us, we will have a better chance. Unfor-
> tunately, a lot of professionals are terrified to do that. Just
> terrified—and for good reason. They are kind of on the out-
> side. They walk a tightrope. The unique ones that I admire
> and who have affected me so positively and affected so
> many others positively, well, they really aren't well re-
> warded by their profession. In fact, I've seen professionals
> lose their jobs for being too honest about how close their
> own personal experiences are to ours.

While respondents can see that professionals are people
like them, who have problems and, in addition, often feel powerless in the face of authority, they did not recognize what, I
would argue, is another similarity. Even as respondents
lamented the professional tendency to stereotype them as a single faceless and falsely homogenous category, when given the
opportunity, consumers and survivors stereotype professionals

in much the same fashion. In addition, "good" mental health professionals, who were seen as having provided real help, didn't appear to be part of any category at all and, for all intents and purposes, slipped quietly off stage while the "us" versus "them" battle raged. Indeed, throughout the study, helpful mental health professionals did not figure into respondents' conversations in any substantial way, unless brought forward as an example of the rare exception that served to prove the rule. This lack of acknowledgement blinds consumers and survivors to a potential source of allies for their cause and, in addition, pre-empts a possibly fruitful discussion about what, exactly, delineates "good" and helpful professionals from their supposedly "bad" and unhelpful colleagues. It also ignores the reality that good professionals, just like their bad colleagues, can have their own entrepreneurial agendas for change which may or may not agree with consumer and survivor goals. Cassin (1993) concludes that defining the category of Other as a uniform and often unattractive "they" is part and parcel of the politics of activism, but the mutual tendency to stereotype can militate against the identification of positive opportunities for co-operation and collaboration between the powerful and the less powerful.

The system

De Certeau (1984) argues that it has been the project of sociology to examine those aspects of human experience which have not been "tamed and symbolized in language" (p. 61). People's everyday lives are full of activities and relationships which, if they are pressed for an explanation, seem best described as "the way things are." There are many instances when "we do not know what it is that we know" (p. 63). In the preceding chapter, consumers and survivors described a process by which they came to "see" and "know" themselves in a new way. In de Certeau's terms, they had discovered the language to describe that which they knew but could not say.

In this vein, there is an expression that continues to crop up, and with such frequency that it seems to demand explanation, yet none is forthcoming. That expression is "the system." Consumers and survivors describe themselves as still in the system or completely out of the system. They argue for change in the system or, alternatively, suggest that the system should be blown up and replaced with something new. They describe what the system did to them and fear for their peers who are left behind in the system. They fight the system, they complain about the system, they advocate from within the system, they reject the system and they blame the system. Consumers and survivors are not alone. Mental health professionals also use the term, and with at least equivalent frequency. We work in the system, we support the system, we advocate on behalf of the system, we rebel against the system, we reform the system, we talk about getting out of the system and, like consumers and survivors, we blame the system.

What is the system? In Janeway's terms, it is a reified metaphor for the power contract. It is the relationship between "us" and "them" and, as such, it is an extremely difficult thing to see and to know because *we* are *it*. In order to know and to see the system, de Certeau suggests what he calls an old recipe, whereby a specific example is "cut out" from the surrounding cloth of the larger, more opaque concept and "made to talk" (1984, pp. 62-63). The example I have chosen to begin to know and see the system is Cedar Glen.

Hugh Tapping was the only respondent who mentioned Cedar Glen. He attended the inquest. Usually, when a subject is raised only once in a study, it is assigned small importance because qualitative data analysis techniques depend heavily on uncovering themes and commonalities among the majority of respondents' experiences. Occasionally, however, just one instance is revealing and demands a place of its own in the research story. Cedar Glen is a case in point.

In 1984, Jean Thibault and his wife Mary Jane purchased a boarding home called Cedar Glen for $250,000 from the Dyke family who, after 15 years in the business, had decided that they wanted a change. It was, by all accounts, an attractive, well-run home for 27 ex-mental patients, most discharged from two provincial psychiatric hospitals, the former Queen Street Mental Health Centre in Toronto and the Penetanguishene Mental Health Centre in Orillia. The house was located in a small village called Uptergrove, not far from Orillia and about 200 kilometres north of Toronto. Not long after the purchase, the public health department and the fire marshal noticed that the home had begun to deteriorate, failing its health and safety inspections three years running because of violations such as locked fire doors and well water contaminated with fecal coliform bacteria (*OPSAnews #2*, 1990).

The condition of the residents was not, however, a matter for concern until May of 1985, when a former Queen Street patient, Ron Eaton, "escaped," as he was later to describe it. Somehow, he made his way back to Toronto and Queen Street Mental Health Centre where he told the Patient Advocate Office that he had been beaten by the owner, Mr. Thibault. A subsequent medical examination showed that he had sustained two broken bones. The institution's advocates contacted the Ontario Provincial Police in Orillia repeatedly, 23 times to be exact, but the officers professed themselves to be powerless to take action due to what they felt was the lack of credibility of the witness (*Inquest*, 1990). In December of the same year, a second resident, 56-year-old Jean Smith, was rushed to hospital covered in bruises and suffering from a severe head injury that resulted in an 11-month-long coma. At this point, the police reconsidered their earlier position and charged Thibault with two counts of assault, allowing bail only on the condition that he stay away from Cedar Glen ("Home's Owner Jailed," 1988). Queen Street staff also visited the home to ask the remaining residents if they wanted to be moved, but they said no, they were fine. Staff concluded that, given that Cedar Glen was a privately owned home, they were powerless to remove the residents unless they clearly stated that they wanted to leave. Later, Pam Dyke, the former owner, was quoted as saying, "[Thibault] supplies you with your food, with your every necessity of life. And he threatens you that if you don't say you want to stay. . . . What are you going to say?" (*W5*, 1988, p. 6).

In the summer of 1987, Doreen and Randy McCunn, as new graduates of the social service program at a nearby community college, sought employment at Cedar Glen and were deeply disturbed by what they witnessed. Thibault, in violation of his bail order, had continued to visit the home, often in a drunken rage. The McCunns witnessed Thibault, his wife Mary Jane and their teenage daughter regularly beat and verbally humiliate residents. They were locked out of doors in winter, clad in very little clothing. The bathrooms were barred at night and residents were punched and kicked when they urinated on the floor. The few residents who tried feebly to escape were returned and beaten. A broomstick was used to batter the testicles of one of the men. Women were forced to sit on chairs while Thibault hit them repeatedly in the face. The heat was turned so low in winter that the residents constantly shivered while the Thibaults wore coats indoors. Food was rationed and the residents often went hungry. Heavy doses of psychiatric medication, prescribed by a local doctor, were administered twice daily, often by the Thibaults' teenage daughter ("Life in Orillia's House of Horrors," 1988). Welfare and old age pension cheques were seized in their entirety, leaving the residents with nothing. The Thibaults' annual income was reported at $156,000 and, in just three years, they amassed enough profit from the operation of Cedar Glen to purchase a separate home on a 110-acre farm, complete with barns, cattle, farm machinery, several cars and a swimming pool (*W5*, 1988).

When the McCunns tried to arrange an interview with the Ministry of Health so that they could reveal what they knew, they got nowhere (*OPSAnews #2*, 1990). They persisted for three months and eventually went to the press in frustration. *W5*, a well-known public affairs television program, agreed to look into the story. Coincidentally, the Ministry of Health and Queen Street staff decided to take action at the exact same moment. They notified the families of the residents that Thibault had been convicted of the assault charges against him, but some had already read about it in the newspaper. Then, on New Year's Eve in 1987, Queen Street staff, accompanied by a Ministry of Health bureaucrat, removed the residents from the home whether they said they wanted to go or not. *W5* cameras recorded the scene as part of a television show called *House of Horrors* that went to air in January 1988.

Unfortunately, these actions came too late for Joseph Kendall, a former Queen Street patient who died, ostensibly from a blood clot on the brain, a month and a half before the *W5* cameras arrived. When the police ordered his body exhumed, it was discovered that the death certificate had been inaccurate. When admitted to hospital, Kendall had been suffering from pneumonia, malnutrition, dehydration and a reaction to overmedication, but what actually killed him was a massive pulmonary embolism due to post-operative complications when surgeons had attempted to repair a hip fracture sustained in an altercation at Cedar Glen (*Inquest*, 1990). Soon afterward, Thibault, his wife and teenage daughter were charged with various counts of assault, and, in September 1989, Thibault received a three-and-a-half-year prison sentence while his wife was sentenced to four months. The daughter, as a juvenile, was placed on probation ("Cedar Glen Home Fallout," 1990).

Joseph Kendall's death was the subject of the longest inquest in Ontario's history, running for four months in late 1990 ("Report Concludes," 1992). Held in Orillia, there was relatively little publicity although the local paper picked up the story and followed it through to its conclusion. Several family members sued Queen Street Mental Health Centre, an individual staff member, the Ministry of Health, the Ministry of Community and Social Services and a second individual social worker who worked for adult protection services in the Orillia area ("Cedar Glen Home Fallout," 1990). The charge was that Queen Street staff and other government officials had known about the abuse but had failed to take action to protect the residents. The suit was eventually settled out of court for an undisclosed amount of money (Barry Swadron, personal communication, October 25, 1994).

However, the conclusion of the coroner's jury was that no one person or set of persons could be held accountable for the Cedar Glen tragedy. While the jury expressed itself to be "shocked and appalled" that such a thing could occur in Canada, its verdict was that it was "the system" that had failed Joseph Kendall and his fellow residents. The jury's recommendations covered every professional group, agency and body that had been involved as the sad story unfolded. Among the lengthy list was a call for a number of new laws, some of which were designed to force professionals to report abuse. Another set was to create a system whereby individual advocates must be assigned to "vulnerable adults" to see that their rights were not violated, and a suggested third set of laws was to focus on the licensing of boarding homes so they could be regulated by government staff. In short, the jury accepted the contention that the many professionals who knew about the conditions at Cedar Glen, yet who had failed to take action, were indeed powerless. Instead of individual culpability, it was the system that was judged to be at fault ("Fight Not Over Yet," 1989). Consequently, the solution was cast in terms of more laws and more staff to enforce them. Remarkably, the jury's recommendations were swiftly and thoroughly acted upon. A commission to look into unregulated housing was immediately appointed, and a report called "A Community of Interest" was released in June 1992 ("Lengthy Inquest Examined Plight," 1991). It formed the basis of Bill 120, which was designed to extend the rights of tenants under the Landlord and Tenant Act so that they also applied to vulnerable adults in unregulated housing. In December of the same year, the Advocacy Act[1] was passed, calling for the establishment of a $23 million commission employing 130 professional advocates ("Report Concludes," 1992). At the same time, the Substitute Decisions Act and the Consent to Treatment Act were also passed ("Handicapped Gain New Voice," 1992; "System Goes Too Far," 1992) and, although complex, both were designed to "expand the rights of adults who are mentally incapable" (*A Guide to the Substitute Decisions Act*, 1994, p. 6).

When Hugh Tapping speaks privately of Cedar Glen, he assigns blame and names names. His memory of the inquest is filled with files suddenly gone missing, inexplicably poor memories and a general look of terror on the faces of the professionals who testified. However, in an article published in *OPSAnews* #2 (1990), he is more reticent.

---

1 One of the first tasks of the newly elected Conservative government was the repeal of the Advocacy Act in March of 1996. In addition, the Substitute Decisions Act and the Consent to Treatment Act were combined into the Health Care Consent Act which, in essence, wiped out the expanded rights and obligations called for by these two separate pieces of legislation ("Tories Move to Repeal," 1995).

> It would be easy to blame the Ministry of Health for what went on at Cedar Glen. . . . It would be easy, and it would be wrong. There are Cedar Glens in every province and state on this continent. The level of violence was the only unique thing about this particular one. (*OPSAnews #2*, 1990, p. 9)

Jennifer Chambers, speaking of instances like Cedar Glen and other examples of what she terms "cowardice in action," points out that everyone has something they fear losing. She says,

> Everybody's afraid. With service providers, it's obvious. They're afraid of losing their jobs. With people who still rely on mental health services, they are afraid that what little they have will be taken from them. People say, "If there's abuse going on, why don't we hear about it?" In the hospital, it's obvious why patients are afraid of complaining. It's like domestic abuse . . . well, in some ways, it's worse. For someone to complain about someone they're living with takes an extraordinary amount of courage, but when people can be involuntarily returned to the institution they may have complained against, there's reason to be terrified.

Schwartz (1994) states that when bad things happen in "the system," the typical government response is to create more rules and regulations because it is the only thing that it knows how to do. Certainly, the uniform rationale among those who had knowledge of the plight of the residents of Cedar Glen was that they were powerless to intervene because there were no laws that allowed residents to be removed from a privately owned home if they were unable to say specifically that they wanted to go. However, as Mrs. Dyke, the former owner countered, why didn't government and hospital staff have the empathy and wisdom to understand that the residents couldn't openly defy the violent Thibaults? Why didn't the moral imperative supersede the legal one? Alice Miller (1984) answers: she states that it is the well-raised child, the obedient and compliant child, who is in particular danger of abandoning autonomous thought and action in favour of the sanctioned path of rules and regulations. In adulthood, these children may attain Wartenberg's (1990) social shell of outward power, composed of university degrees, important jobs and respected titles. However, when tested, it is the child's remembered sense of powerlessness that surfaces, evoking feelings of danger and vulnerability, overwhelming independent judgement. To do as one is told is the price of membership within the universe of obligation, and, when there is no rule to follow, the safest course of action is to do nothing.

There is a curious silence among consumers and survivors regarding Cedar Glen. Many simply don't know about it, but this in itself is odd, given that a detailed report, sparing none of the ugliness, was published in a widely circulated survivor-generated newsletter (*OPSAnews #2*, 1990). Cedar Glen offers the clearest, publicly acknowledged and most thoroughly negative portrait of "them" available, yet it has not been embraced as a plank in the activists' platform. Certainly, the legislative flurry that followed the incident entailed the enactment of laws that consumers and survivors had previously only dreamed possible. However, laws are blunt instruments, and Hugh Tapping concludes his article on Cedar Glen with a note of discomfort which had seemingly begun to sound in his mind. He says, "Legislation can make it easier for people to do their jobs. But how can a law make people care?" (*OPSAnews #2*, 1990, p. 9).

There is the possibility that what happened at Cedar Glen offers more "knowing" and "seeing" than is palatable for consumers and survivors. If "they" are afraid and "we" are afraid, who's in charge? Some respondents believe that the system represents a power contract that can never work. Donna says, "It's my hope that people will figure out that there's nothing here, that professionals talking to you and reading books and taking counselling courses can't change what's in your mind." Chamberlin (1978), a long-time proponent of self-help and survivor-run alternatives to the formal system, agrees. But there are others who, like Jane Pritchard, say, "if they would just do their jobs. . . ."

The paradox of Other, the reflecting mirror that defines that which we are *not*, is that it assumes an intimate relationship between subject and object, one which is, at one and the same time, adversarial (they behave badly) yet infused with hope (they don't *really* mean it). The process of empowerment is one of letting go of expectations, bitterness and anger, and refocusing energy on enhancing self-capacity and fashioning an independent future (Gadacz, 1994). However, consumers and survivors are in a curious position. Many remain entwined in the services offered by the mental health system by virtue of their need for social assistance and affordable housing. Others are active consumers of medication, counselling and group therapy. They need what mental health professionals have to offer and although some will, as Donna hopes, give up on the system, while others will toil to create their own alternative services, most cannot exit the power contract that they claim is not working. As a result, developing a clear, unequivocal definition of who their social movement's "enemy" is becomes a circular, emotional and complex debate.

In conclusion

The Scottish poet Robbie Burns wished that God could grant us the gift to see ourselves as others see us. He was probably alone in this. Most of us have no desire to hear the unvarnished opinions of "us" offered by "them." Consumers and survivors typically enter the mental health system through the doors of psychiatric hospitals where it is routine and in fact de rigueur for professionals to offer written and verbal assessments of them. My own experience taught me that we tend to see patients as sick, manipulative, non-compliant, unmotivated, ungrateful, hopeless and helpless. When the tables are turned, and consumers and survivors are in a position to offer their assessments of us, they judge us to be willfully deaf and blind, emotionally constricted, misguided at best, abusive at worst and, when threatened, sycophantic and cowardly. In addition, they say that we disguise our own vulnerabilities and despise the very help we are supposed to be giving. The system, as the place where "we" and "they" interact, seems to make us all, as Jennifer Chambers says, afraid: afraid of losing our jobs, afraid of losing what little we have, afraid of saying what we think and afraid to tell. However, as the next chapter reveals, consumers and survivors are as hard on each other as they are on mental health professionals.

7

Us

As consumers and survivors continue to find one another and share their common experiences and grievances, they are challenged with the task of formalizing their association. Gamson (1991) believes that any group or movement that wants a continued commitment from its membership must construct a collective identity—consumers and survivors must become an acknowledged "us" which is demonstrably different from "them." Implicit in a collective identity is a sense of solidarity—group members must hang together so they don't hang separately, as Janeway (1980) puts it. Chamberlin (1978, 1990) is adamant that self-help is the most natural rallying point for consumers and survivors and, indeed, these sorts of groups are an excellent breeding ground for social activism (Gamson, 1991).

The Canadian document *Framework for Support of People with Severe Disabilities* (Trainor & Church, 1984) identified self-help as only one component in the construction of an appropriate mental health system and, by virtue of its central theme—a redefinition of the mental patient as citizen rather than service recipient—tended to concentrate its emphasis on a call for a central role for newly named consumers in the planning, development and delivery of all mental health services. This publication was quietly received until it was put to the test during the consultation process that led to the Graham Report (Graham, 1988), precursor to the formal government policy document called *Putting People First* (1993). At that time, consumers and survivors became intensely involved with professionals under the rubric of *participation*. Consequently, in Ontario, any discussion of the development of a group identity for consumers and survivors must be played out against the backdrop of the hovering presence of "them"—mental health professionals, bureaucrats and other government figures.

Getting involved

Susan Marshall, who told her story in chapter 5, said that when she realized that she wasn't alone in her experience of the psychiatric system, she began to get angry. However, for many respondents, the journey from ex-mental patient to consumer or survivor is an assisted one, in that very often mental health professionals were involved in some fashion. A respondent who wished to remain anonymous explains:

> Mine is kind of a funny story. I never thought of myself as a consumer/survivor or had any kind of identity like that. But, at the Employment Office, I saw something put up by a local Toronto agency. They were looking for a project manager who was familiar with issues around personnel and human resources, and someone who had knowledge of the mental health system. I had no concept of consumer/survivor. I thought I was just a fuck-up ... just couldn't get it together. A failure, right? And so anyway, just for a joke, I fired off this resume and I said that I would discuss my knowledge of the mental health system with them in person. Well, they called me for an interview and they said, "What about your knowledge of the mental health system?" And I kind of laughed to myself because I didn't think they would want *my* kind of experience but I answered anyway. And one of the guys interviewing me said, "You're a consumer/survivor." Fortunately, the meaning of the term was kind of obvious to me, so I said, "Yeah, yeah. That's what I am." So a mental health agency made me a consumer/survivor. Now, there's a turn of events!

While this respondent identifies her recruitment by a mental health agency as unique, she is in no way alone. In fact, mental health professionals were typically instrumental, directly or indirectly, in respondents' participation. Given the emphasis on partnership that had, by the time of my research, enshrined itself formally in Ministry of Health evaluation procedures for mental health programs and agencies, it is not really surprising that professionals played such a prominent role in consumer and survivor recruitment. Yet, respondents typically described it as something that happened "just by accident."

Others pointed to a government-sponsored conference called Our Turn, held in Montreal in November 1989, as particularly transforming. Adele Rosenbloom helped organize the event. She is a 39-year-old mother of two boys and a self-described Jewish feminist activist who started having problems at a point in her life when she began identifying as a lesbian, a lifestyle that her mother disapproved of. Because she worked in a group home run by a feminist collective, she was able to rely on her co-workers for support and assistance during her most difficult periods, but her mother felt that treatment from the formal mental health system was in order. She suggested that Adele accompany her to a hospital with the promise that a psychiatrist whom Adele had found to be helpful would meet them there. However, once they arrived, it was revealed that it had all been a trick to get her admitted. Frightened and angry, Adele tried to run, but she was picked up by the police, certified by the duty doctor, restrained and given Haldol by injection. She was held for 11 days on a psychiatric ward. Adele says:

> It was after that experience that I got involved in organizing the Our Turn conference. Survivors from all across Canada came together with funding from the government and we had a wonderful time. We met in Montreal for about five days and, really, that whole event was so empowering and liberating. I felt truly supported and understood. I came away feeling strong and I lost a lot of the shame that I felt as a result of being locked up. For me, it helped build self-esteem again.

Dave Stewart, staff to the Patient Council in a psychiatric hospital in the eastern part of the province, also attended the conference. Dave describes himself as a problem kid—the "black sheep" of the family. "I had no self-worth, no self-

esteem. My family had already disowned me, emotionally anyway, and I was experiencing great bouts of depression. Suicide
was an obvious way out." Hospitalization, to Dave, meant being
put away for the rest of his life. But, as he says, "I was a bad
patient," so he was let out. His experience of the Our Turn conference was intense, demonstrating for the first time, that he
wasn't alone.

For other respondents, their formal involvement as a participant came when they were hired by one of the many newly
funded Consumer/Survivor Development Initiative (CSDI) projects. Paul Reeve says that he saw an ad in the paper and he was
amazed. "Here was a job where you *had* to be an ex-mental
patient to qualify and all you had to do was declare it." Louise
St. Jacques, writing in the *OPSAnews #7* (1992), echoes Paul's
surprise: "I never dreamed that being labelled crazy would land
me a job." Donna adds that, in fact, she had never thought of
herself as a consumer until a job came up that listed direct
experience of the mental health system as a requirement.
Susan Marshall, as well, credits a job as the impetus for her
involvement. And, as Paul indicates, all people had to do to
compete for the 300[1] mostly part-time jobs that were originally
created through CSDI was to declare that they were ex-mental
patients.

Certainly, these sorts of opportunities afforded those who
chose to "go public" the possibility of a new and more valued
social role: as "partners," or, as it is often termed, "stakeholders" instead of marginalized ex-mental patients. Participation
also meant that consumers and survivors began to have a substantial presence in the mental health system due to the kind
of power that sheer numbers can provide. Indeed, CSDI funding
created consumer- and survivor-controlled projects all over the
province and each could be said to equal what Berger (1977)
calls a mediation structure—a mid-sized organization or association that serves as a bridge between the individual and the
large institutions of society. In fact, the CSDI programs became
visible recruitment pools to which mental health professionals

---

1 In 1995, these numbers had shrunk to 161 employed in 36 CSDI projects
province-wide (Dewar, 1995).

and government bureaucrats could turn when seeking stake-holders for the many activities related to mental health reform. The new demand that consumers and survivors sit side by side with professionals and bureaucrats as they planned changes in mental health services signalled a substantial shift in the traditional power contract between these groups. Participation also afforded large numbers of ex-mental patients an opportunity for influence which historically had only been achieved through the precarious authority of the lone-wolf advocate. However, some respondents reported that "going public" was a heavy price to pay for their new-found status. Mary offers her thoughts:

> The doctor I was seeing was really supportive and helped me weigh the pros and cons of going public. Now, I kind of regret . . . like, what did I do by letting people know I was a consumer? It's blocked all these avenues for me. . . . A lot of times, because of the amount of funding for consumer projects, especially in Ontario, people have just jumped in with both feet because they could get a paying job by revealing they were a consumer or a psychiatric survivor. Sometimes they haven't even thought through the implications.

Susan Marshall feels that she has been able to handle the stigma, but her small daughter has been affected. She says, "There are a few of her playmates who are no longer allowed to come to our house." Marnie Shepherd, a survivor herself, feels that life in a small town can be especially difficult for self-identified consumers and survivors. She says:

> I work with a group that, when they looked for office space, it couldn't be on the main street. It's a small community and everybody knows when you go in that door where you are going. So they're off the main street and they're in a small building that has some other services in it that aren't related to mental health so people can come in. In rural Ontario, consumer/survivors struggle with the stigma.

The issue of stigma aside, some respondents seemed embarrassed to admit that their sensitization to the consumer and survivor movement came about because of a job, indicating that it wasn't quite a pure-enough motivation. In fact, 11 out of the study's 13 employed respondents were working for some sort of government-funded consumer and survivor project—most of which were sponsored through the Consumer/Survivor Development Initiative—and an additional 3 had worked previously for such programs. In fact, CSDI funded a total of 42 advocacy or economic development projects across the province in the first few months of operation. This level of activity represents a clear demonstration of the impact of government funding on consumer and survivor activism.

Gamson (1995) states that it is not uncommon for groups who have been excluded from society's universe of obligation to have their fate reversed. For literally centuries, no one has much cared what mental patients thought or believed. However, in the early 1990s, the Ontario government seemed to have begun to care deeply and, as a measure of good intention, assigned a small dollar figure (in the overall scheme of things) to demonstrate its good will. The governmental view of consumers and survivors is rife with those sorts of paradoxes that merit close attention. In one set of laws, it endorses a *parens patriae* philosophy, providing the legal avenue for suspending the civil rights of people who are judged to be mentally ill. On the other hand, it actively recruits these same mentally ill people to participate in the production of public policy. Although it is a large question, the notion of why now? requires some consideration. One clue may be that consumers and psychiatric survivors are typically critical of professionally dominated mental health services, particularly psychiatrists and institutions—the more costly components of the health care system. Continually rising costs require countervailing measures based on a logic that taxpayers can assimilate as reasonable justification for either capping expenditures or cutting back. Customer dissatisfaction is a saleable rationale for downsizing the institutionally based portion of the mental health system and modifying the rest. Also, consumers and survivors tend to advocate most strongly for really cheap things such as self-help and economic development projects and, as a result, these sorts of alternatives enjoyed a new emphasis in formal government policies such as *Putting People First*. In addition, they are supportive of less-expensive community-based, non-institutional services because it is with these types of programs that essentials such as housing are offered.

Pressures such as fiscal restraint, along with a general reduction in admiration for experts and an increased emphasis on prosumerism (Toffler, 1990) combined with the utility of a consumer dissatisfaction logic, provide a synchronicity of motives that, speculatively, may offer at least a portion of the answer to the question of why, now, some consumers and survivors are enjoying at least a symbolic reversal in their typically marginalized status. A further point that merits mention is the recent availability of a socially valued political activist role for ex-patients. This new role has provided the means whereby former patients can remain involved in the mental health system. Historically, their choices were twofold: stay as a sick and shunned service recipient or get well and get out, all the while taking steps to disguise a shameful past.

However, Dianna Capponi (1992), in a keynote address at a CSDI conference, argued that this new role, coupled with sudden popularity, was not as enjoyable as it may have seemed. Instead, it had sapped the energy from a nascent social movement, preventing it from developing the strength that a slow, step-by-step evolution would provide while, at the same time, redirecting much-needed humanpower and very scarce emotional resources towards eternal wrangling with government bureaucrats over funding issues and other complaints related to the mechanics of funding.

Is this a social movement?

I thought it important to ask the study's respondents if they felt that what was happening among consumers and survivors had the weight of a social movement in the same way that the peace, women's or environmental movements are. Their answer was "maybe." Marilyn Nearing says:

> I think that consumers and survivors feel that they have been vulnerable and have suffered a kind of stigma which is every bit as strong as racial prejudice. I think all prejudice is tantamount to being labelled and overgeneralized and I think we're rebelling in almost the same way. We're saying, "Look at me as an individual, value me as an individ-

ual"—which is about what every social movement has been founded on.

But Sue Goodwin adds:

> Nobody knows what a consumer or a survivor is. If I go around saying I'm a consumer, they think I work for Consumers Distributing. And if I say I'm a survivor, people say, "Survivor of what?" The truth is that nobody in the whole wide world understands what a consumer or a survivor is.

John (who preferred to be identified only by a pseudonym) adds:

> I'm not sure if you could say it's a social movement because, although there are some isolated pockets of people doing things, I think there must be, what? 95% of the people who are not connected with activism or don't have the resources to do anything like that. A lot of them are just too busy surviving. They're busy from day to day, trying to get food and lodging. They have different interests than the people who have a fairly good quality of life and who have time and health and resources to set up protests. A lot of people feel very powerless.

Patrick Brown looks at it from another angle. He feels, as Alvin Toffler does, that society itself has changed. It is now ready for a new kind of activism.

> I think it came out of society becoming more aware of the fact that not every consumer/survivor fits the image of the typical stereotype like somebody walking down the street barefoot, eating out of a garbage can. I think society has realized that survivors or consumer/survivors, whatever term you want to use, are people who probably had a breakdown once in their life and recovered and can make a contribution. Vincent van Gogh had a mental illness. Winston Churchill, too, and the list goes on. It's a natural social process. It's not something that was pushed ahead by any one group of people.

Jane Pritchard is more pessimistic. She says, "By virtue of the fact that we have a common bond, a common experience, we have a movement but we haven't gotten our shit together, to be perfectly honest and blunt about it." Jennifer Reid agrees.

> This movement is thousands strong but we're not united and, until we are, we're not going anywhere. If we were united, we could stop Yonge Street. We could just sit down and say, "No! We don't want this crap anymore." But we won't do it. We're afraid of losing our jobs, or afraid that the government will stop our welfare cheques. We're afraid of losing our housing and of going back into hospital. And we're afraid that if we're known as a political agitator, we'll get held in hospital longer.

These comments seem to indicate that, while there are definitely shared experiences and grievances among respondents, they feel that they have not developed the kind of solidarity that other movements enjoy. However, there is some evidence that they have, at least, *begun* to form a movement. For example, during the early days of reform, the Ontario government and mental health professionals in general recognized them individually and collectively, formally and informally, even if motives were tangled. Second, their newly acquired access to previously forbidden territory such as Boards of Directors, task forces and government committees has increased their potential for influence exponentially. In fact, their simple presence in places and situations where professionals and bureaucrats used to confer in private has forced a shift in the nature of the traditional power contract. A prime source of evidence for this shift lies in the language changes that characterized mental health reform rhetoric and writing, an example of which is the use of the term "survivor" in government policies and documents, a definitive, politicized acknowledgement. However, study respondents seem unable to recognize these effects. One reason may be that the changes they envision are so much greater than these largely symbolic victories that it's hard to celebrate so little when so much remains to be accomplished. Certainly, Jennifer Chambers states that it's very difficult "retaining focus in the face of the overwhelming number of things that need doing." Additionally, consumers and survivors have a heightened sense of urgency that drives their desire for change. Having "been there," they contend that their peers are dying while planning exercises go on and on (Church, 1996). This sense of immediacy makes honouring small incremental gains

difficult. Further, having become accustomed to seeing the
world from the bottom-up position of marginalization rather
than the top-down position of system planning, consumers and
survivors have little faith in words, viewing concrete action as
the only solid evidence that real change is underway. Given
their heavily stigmatized public identities outside the narrow
world of mental heath reform, combined with the extreme
paucity of their monetary, emotional and human resources,
consumers and survivors are coming from a starting position
which could be said to be far behind that of members of other
movements. While involvement in government committees and
agency Boards may offer some reward, the reality is that many
consumers' and survivors' lives remain characterized by
poverty, unstable housing, unemployment and the possibility
that they may, once again, find themselves in the very institutions they have so vociferously attacked. In this latter situation,
their newly acquired power and status doesn't go merely unap-
preciated—it becomes a potential threat to their safety.

Consumer? Survivor? Consumer/survivor? Or just a person?

So far in this work, I have been careful to use both
consumer and psychiatric survivor when speaking of respondents. I have also occasionally thrown in the hybrid version, con-
sumer/survivor. Church (1992) states that this latter term was
invented for a paper entitled "Doing the right* thing right"
(1990), co-authored with David Reville, a prominent ex-mental
patient activist and former Member of the Provincial Parlia-
ment. While terms such as consumer or psychiatric survivor
may appear to be simply a utilitarian way to communicate the
changed status of ex-mental patients, in reality, each designation has a loyal following in a hotly contested political identity
debate.

The naming of oneself or one's group is a political act,
because "domination and colonization attempt to destroy our
capacity to know the self, to know who we are" (hooks, 1989,
p. 31). Mental patients have typically had their identities
defined by mental health professionals—being "labelled" as

some consumers and survivors call it—who have acquired the term from Thomas Scheff's (1966) work on labelling theory. Labels are psychiatric diagnoses: schizophrenia, manic-depression, borderline personality disorder and so on. However, psychiatric diagnoses are prone to becoming an enveloping identity (Estroff, 1989). In addition to these formal labels, mental health professionals often call mental patients other things, such as manipulative, unmotivated, ungrateful and non-compliant. And, finally, the general public has a variety of names: crazies, nutbars, looney toons, weirdos and psychos.

In chapter 5, Marg Oswin states that she believes that mental patients experience a unique form of oppression when the site of colonization is the mind, one that reduces them to nothingness—a cipher, as she calls it. The special bond that is created out of this experience has inspired ex-mental patients to reclaim and name their own identity so that they can, at one and the same time, capture the uniqueness of their oppression and reject vehemently other people's labels. The construction of a political identity is a complex matter in our present-day social world, where there are a multiplicity of choices available related to people's membership in a variety of different collec-tivities (Moghadam, 1994). Certainly, gender, race or ethnicity are irreducible sources of identity (Aronowitz, 1992), but, beyond these visible characteristics, people may choose the level of emphasis they wish to accord other group loyalties. The purpose, however, of creating an identity is to produce an "us" with a shared history and belief system (Papanek, 1994; Smith, 1994). *Consumer*, as discussed in chapter 4, is a designation that grew out of literature that focuses on the rights of mental patients as citizens. It is a rather mild-mannered term that attempts to empower patients and clients by equating them with customers—a term which, in the sphere of the market-place, denotes people who are respected because they demand satisfaction or else they take their business elsewhere.

On the other hand, psychiatric survivor, with its much more in-your-face connotation, was coined by ex-mental patients themselves. It is intended to convey strength in the face of adversity, a sense of optimism and independence, and, above all, power. Without exception, this study's respondents identified themselves as survivors. Consumer was considered a term that was "imposed by the government," according to Sue Goodwin. Walter Osoka adds, "Consumer means that you actually buy it." Indeed, this was the most common view of who a consumer is—someone who consorts willingly with the enemy without benefit of the political analyses that survivors have developed. Jennifer Chambers adds, "consumers tend to be people who believe in mental illness while survivors look more at the social causes of people's distress." Consumer also means dependence. Patrick Brown states: "They depend on the system for the rest of their lives. From the day they get sick to the day they die, they're consuming services. That's what a true consumer is." Another respondent felt that the standard marketplace meaning of consumer simply doesn't apply in this case.

> It suggests that there's this huge psychiatric shopping mall where you can go and pick your services. So, it implies a choice when actually the choice is very limited and, in some cases, there is no choice at all. And the second reason that I don't like the term is that it suggests that all we do is consume, that we're always taking, where I think that I also contribute something to my community.

Jennifer Reid concludes the discussion succinctly. She says, "I didn't consume the system. The system consumed me."

On the other hand, the term psychiatric survivor had an emotional commitment which was evident in the many sub-meanings that respondents accorded its definition. For example, eight respondents specifically identified themselves as survivors of sexual abuse which, from their perspective, gave psychiatric survivor an intended double meaning—survivor of child abuse and survivor of the mental health system. Marilyn Nearing says, "The prevalence of abuse among members of this movement is extremely high. And I don't any longer take it as a given that all of us do survive—a lot of us haven't. I take great pride in that word and I wear it like a medal."

Indeed, Marilyn is not wrong in her belief that child abuse is a common experience among current and former psychiatric patients. In a review of 8 studies involving 587 female psychiatric patients, findings ranged from 65% to 97% reporting severe child abuse. When sexual abuse alone was examined, the figures ranged from 37% to 65%, indicating an extensive problem (Beck & van der Kolk, 1987; Bryer et al., 1987; Chu & Dill, 1990; Firsten, 1991; Goodman, Dutton & Harris, 1995; Muenzenmaier et al., 1993; Steiner Crane et al., 1988; Zlotnick et al., 1995). Further, in a study of 125 male psychiatric patients (Swett, Surrey & Cohen, 1990), it was reported that 48% had experienced child abuse with 7% reporting sexual abuse, although there is always speculation that men especially underreport sexual abuse due to fears that they might be thought gay or have been caused to be gay (if the abuser was a man) or of ridicule (if the abuser was a woman) (Lew, 1988).

The second aspect of the survivor identity is surviving the system. Jennifer Reid says, "I use the word survivor because the psychiatric system rapes people and, if you get raped, what are you? You're a survivor."

An additional and important meaning was the idea of surviving what *might* have happened—those things that respondents felt they were lucky to have escaped. Donna explains:

> I had a very bad go a few years ago now and I was pretty dysfunctional, but I was married to a man who could afford to support me so when I quit my job because I really couldn't get up in the morning, it was OK. All the things were in place to just let me dwell in my sorrow, if I can put it that way. And I understood from my earlier experiences that if I could just hang on, it would pass. Now, it took a long time, but it did pass and my point is that if I can avoid the system because of my social economic situation, then obviously it's being used for the lepers of today—the throwaways. The whole institution is built around poverty. It's not built around need. The bottom line is that the only thing that saved me happened to be my socio-economic position and that, to me, is terrifying. It was the only difference between what could have been done to me and what wasn't done.

Another respondent who prefers to be identified only as M. echoes Donna's point. She says, "There but for the grace of God go I. Had my birth been different, had my upbringing been different, had my education been different, had my illness been different, I mightn't be where I am today." Thus, while it might be supposed that the survivor identity is acquired only after worst-case examples of involuntary hospitalization, these respondents point out the extremes of discomfort they feel because they are now identified members of a group who *could* be committed. They also worry because poverty and pessimism is the typical condition in which most members of their group live.

Patrick Brown says:

> When I'm down at the hospital where I used to get treatment, I see people that I knew 10 years ago and they're in the same state. They haven't regressed or progressed. That's a wasted life. I'm not better than those people, I want to make that totally clear. It's just that some of the opportunities that I've gotten, those people haven't had.

Patrick goes on to say that he also survived what he calls "the experiment." "Most of us are guinea pigs, let's face it. Right now, there are a lot of drugs in psychiatry and they don't know how they work." Patrick is referring to the kind of specialized information, formerly available exclusively to physicians, that is now reasonably easy for anyone to access. For example, the *Compendium of Canadian Pharmaceuticals*, a highly technical reference written with physicians in mind, can be found in most libraries, and it says very much what Patrick says: it has not yet been discovered how psychiatric medications work in the brain.

Another respondent, in offering her personal definition of psychiatric survivor, tells how she explained it to her family. She says:

> My parents didn't know about my mental health history, right? I got involved in the system after I ran away from home. So, when I go home now, they're always remarking on my job at the centre saying, "You're so great to work with 'those' people." And I couldn't stand it any longer so I said, "Look, I'm one of those people." Well, my mother just kind of shut down but my father said, "Who told you that?" So I went through the whole consumer/survivor explanation. So he says, "Ahh, in this country"—he's not from Canada—"in this country, as soon as you stand up and say something, they tell you you're crazy. You shouldn't call yourselves that. You should call yourselves 'people who

know what's really going on.'" So that's his take on the whole thing.

Finally, Walter Osoka offers a definition that just about covers the waterfront. He says, "Being a survivor means surviving mental health services, surviving the help we were supposed to get, surviving the stigma, the side effects of the medications, the loneliness, hunger, homelessness, abuse, the illness itself and surviving losing your rights as a citizen."

The hybrid version, consumer/survivor, invented by Reville and Church (1990), figured prominently in respondents' conversations, but it appeared to have been adopted as a convenience term as well as a form of bridging language for occasions when both groups, psychiatric survivors and professionals, work together. It is the term used in *Putting People First*, and it can be found in a variety of other government documents. However, from the perspective of many respondents, the official sanction of the term consumer/survivor appears to have sapped the shock value from "psychiatric survivor" while, at the same time, politicized by association the tamer version, "consumer." Church (1992) herself says that it seems to have stilled, rather than encouraged, debate. Whatever the case, Sue Goodwin says that she's not fooled by any of it.

> The government invented the whole thing. It's supposed to be kinder than calling us ex-psychiatric patients. It's also for people in the movement who object to being called consumers because no one knows what the fuck that is and it's for people who don't want to be called survivors because then people will know that you're a scary mental patient. So they put a slash in between the two things so we wouldn't have an identity crisis.

Indeed, some members of the survivor group feel that their identity has been stolen once again and, in a variety of Internet exchanges, have begun calling themselves crazies or lunatics in an effort to retain a radical edge.

The adoption of a political activist identity, whether consumer or survivor, offers respondents a less-stigmatized status than ex-mental patient and, as a consequence, access to power and influence previously denied them. However, as Sue Goodwin points out, its utility is virtually non-existent outside the small world of mental health and mental health services. Jane Pritchard talks about how narrow the world can become if all possible identities are divided between consumer and survivor. She says:

> I don't want to just survive. I want to thrive. But even that's silly. If I asked you, Barbara, who you were, you wouldn't say you were a "survivor" or a "thriver" or anything like that. And if I meet friends or family or anyone who's not connected with the mental health system, then I certainly don't describe myself as any of those things. I'm just a person.

Among this set of respondents, the term "consumer" was rejected outright as their choice for an identity. As Marg Oswin says, "there's an interpretation that consumers are soft survivors, tentative survivors, future survivors." There are also much stronger opinions. Hurst (1990) says, "Consumers exist but survivors succeed. . . . A consumer gives in to advertising, to pressure, and to the wishes of [service] providers. A survivor has fought, endured and triumphed, like a survivor of Auschwitz" (p. 7).

The intense and sometimes acrimonious struggle over these two identities suggests the possibility of the presence of two minds within the individual activists. Certainly, none of the study's respondents was prepared to deny that they had experienced serious problems and had eventually reached out for help, "consuming" mental health services, as it were. John says that the thing with mental illness is that you just never know if it might happen again. Mary confirms this sense of uncertainty. "It's the oscillation between hope and despair that we all go through, but a lot of us are closer to the despairing side and we are seeking hope." M. describes it more fully:

> We are the children of Sisyphus. Sisyphus is a mythological character doomed to an eternity of rolling a heavy stone to the top of a hill and every time it gets to the top, it rolls back down again and he has to roll it back up again—for all eternity. Up and down, up and down. And for many survivors, that's their life. They have their good times and then they'll reach the depths of depression, not able to come out of their room for days or, on the other spinoff, find themselves wildly hallucinating and out of control.

Even Hugh Tapping, an avowed and long-term survivor, repeatedly described himself as "clinically depressed" during his research interview. When I asked him why he was using psychiatric terminology when he clearly rejects that view, he said:

> Calling myself clinically depressed seems clearer than saying I'm fucked up beyond all recognition. It's a short form. I don't think I'm clinically depressed insofar as I'm suffering from a biochemical disorder with some kind of genetic component involving my you-name-it neurotransmitter. I'm hurt and I'm pissed off. Depression and anger, the same thing. Rage at the universe turned inwards. Just because you have all the insight in the world doesn't mean it's necessarily going to help.

In fact, many respondents, in passing, revealed that they still took medication now and again or that they saw a therapist or a psychiatrist so, in terms of everyday reality, the lines between the terms consumer and survivor are much more blurred than in their political iteration. It also points to the likelihood of a competition between the identities of political activist and that of service recipient—a competition that can impede personal empowerment. On one hand, respondents believe that the service recipient role requires them to put up with whatever help they get without complaint while, at the same time, they struggle with developing and maintaining a political identity based on an ongoing and vociferous critique of that self-same help—a difficult balancing act indeed. In addition, it appears that embracing the more strongly politicized psychiatric survivor identity does not insulate people against the fear that they may, one day, need help again. Were this to be the case, where can survivors go? Given their hard-line stance against professionally run mental health services and psychiatric medication, combined with the belief that they may experience retaliation should they find themselves once again in an institution, their options are slim.

When some of "us" joined "them"

While language is an important site of struggle, so, too, is money. When the Consumer/Survivor Development Initiative (CSDI) began operation, it hired five consumer/survivors as staff, and they suddenly joined the ranks of the enemy, so to speak, becoming, essentially, Ministry of Health bureaucrats. However, a professional rather than a consumer was selected to head the program. Susan Marshall says, "God forbid they would get an actual consumer/survivor to run it and make the *real* decisions. The only way they could sell this idea was to have a 'normal' person in there." Dave Stewart agrees: "They couldn't have got the political acceptance even with one of our most prominent leaders at the head." Hugh Tapping is a bit tougher: "The professionals own it. They operate it. If they feel you're out of line, you're gone in two weeks."

The five CSDI consumer/survivors were immediately christened the Dream Team by many of their Toronto peers. The nickname was not intended as a compliment. Instead, it was a reference to a movie of the same name where childlike mental patients, on an outing from a psychiatric institution, are left on their own in a rough part of the city and end up having cute adventures. In other words, the CSDI "Team" was considered to consist of naive dupes hired to parrot the agenda of the professional in charge. Marnie Shepherd, one of the survivor staff members, reflects on this perception of her and her colleagues.

> I spent a lot of time in the first year feeling angry because we'd hear people saying CSDI *was* the professional in charge. I felt a lot of consumer/survivors were doing a disservice to us, assuming that we were just complacent. I was in the job a month when one survivor met with our boss over a beer and told him that he knew why my colleagues and I had been hired. He said it was because the Ministry knew that we were just compliant consumers. If somebody said that about me today, I'd still be hurt but I'd have a tougher skin. At the time, I was devastated. But, I've had more than one person tell me that we were selling out.

The Consumer/Survivor Development Initiative was governed by a number of specially developed Ministry of Health rules that consumer and survivor groups had to follow if they wanted funds. First, the projects could not mimic professional services. Help and support for program members could be provided only through an egalitarian self-help approach—Chamberlin's notion of the most natural rallying point for consumers and survivors. Second, projects had to aim towards independence as soon as possible. This meant that, although they might have been given a home with a professional agency during the start-up phase for administrative purposes, they were to work towards incorporation and the recruitment of their own Boards of Directors as a priority. Third, they were to hire consumers and survivors exclusively, with one or two narrow exceptions. Board and committee members, elected democratically from a general membership, also had to be consumers and survivors, although this last directive has been relaxed. While CSDI rules appeared to have quite thoroughly taken consumer and survivor views and philosophies into account, respondents were critical, remarking that these sorts of stipulations were an authoritarian statement on how the government expected power to be handled in the CSDI projects. Marilyn Nearing says, "They're afraid that we'll get into the same sort of power dynamics that have been perpetuated by the medical model. It's a knee-jerk reaction to the mental health system—a grand experiment." Jennifer Chambers agrees, but adds the point that the CSDI projects simply could not be seen as in competition with professional services. She says, "I had a paid position with one of the projects as a peer counsellor and CSDI cut it. We were never able to get a clear answer as to why, but all the rumours agreed that it was considered threatening to the professionals who did that kind of work." Dave Stewart adds, "I have a feeling that the formal system wouldn't have been supportive of CSDI if the mandate had been anything other than what it was."

Whatever the reasons behind the CSDI philosophy, many groups, some hastily constructed, others with an acknowledged history, succeeded in meeting the qualifications for funding and received what was, relatively speaking, an astounding amount of money. The salaries CSDI was offering were, in fact, attractive by anyone's standards. Many newly employed project staff went from the poverty of social assistance (approximately

$7,000 to $9,000 dollars per year) to quadruple that amount for full-time work. Marnie says:

> I think if I had to do it all over again, I would have advocated for less money the first year because there was just too much and it came so suddenly . . . to go from having no money to a budget of $100,000 and 2 1/2 staff. Literally, a cheque went out with the only instruction being, at the end of the year, to account for how the money was spent and that was it.

Mary says it was all too fast.

> I believe the intent was good, but they were not really working with us at our pace. I just see us needing to come together to decide, who are we? What are we all about? The additional stressors of the dollars coming in . . . we've just been spread way too thin. The bureaucratic and organizational skills are lacking and the few leaders we have spent their time trying to do the administrative work so we couldn't do the leadership development like we should have.

Hugh Tapping is a lot more critical.

> You start off with a naive bunch of people. They don't know how to be members of an organization because they have never been in one before. They're not stupid. They just don't know about these things. And then things don't work out right? . . . shit, we've been broke all these years and finally we got some money and we thought things were going to be wonderful and they weren't.

He is even tougher on the economic development projects funded through CSDI.

> They don't have a snowball's chance in hell. All they know about the business world is what they learned in a sheltered workshop in a "rehabilitation" environment. The vast majority of people talk about wanting to have a real job . . . in the real world, with a real boss and real work to do. If you get paid, you've done your job. If you don't do your job, you get fired . . . that sort of thing. It's not there for your "mental health." It's not there for your "peer self-help." You do a job and get a roof over your head and that's that.

John concludes more positively:

> It's a really good alternative to sitting with a therapist once a week and, in a lot of cases, it's better.

Obviously, despite what appears to have been good intentions, CSDI is not without its detractors. Respondents point to a lack of skills on the part of the groups that received the money, requiring them to struggle with the complexities associated with running a non-profit organization to the neglect of the self-help and advocacy goals that were their founding mandate. Also, many of the burgeoning movement's leaders were diverted from their more ideologically based functions in order to cope with mundane administrative demands. In some cases, the sheer amount of money received was difficult to handle both organizationally and individually. Visible CSDI organizations became redefined as places of recruitment for agencies and psychiatric hospitals who, by Ministry decree, had to have consumers and survivors on their Boards and committees. These sorts of demands meant that some project staff and members were "spread way too thin," as Mary says. Perhaps the most telling result of the CSDI program was that potential solutions to the consumer and survivor community's many problems became defined in terms of money. "More, more, the need is so great" became the familiar and eternal cry, mimicking the common refrain in most mental health professional circles.

While respondents' views on CSDI projects are mixed, it must nevertheless be acknowledged that the programs have been designed for and by consumers and survivors themselves—completely in concert with the long-sought-after acknowledgement of the value of self-help and employment. Also, from a traditional shoestring, self-help perspective, they are generously funded and resourced. While members and staff are struggling, they clearly have the opportunity to learn skills, acquire new knowledge and participate in their communities in ways that have previously been denied.

The Ontario Psychiatric Survivors Alliance

The sorts of tensions and criticisms sparked by CSDI were nowhere more evident than in the provincial organization it funded, the Ontario Psychiatric Survivors Alliance (OPSA). OPSA had a tumultuous and short-lived existence. What exactly happened is hard to determine because consumers and survivors are not terribly comfortable talking about the subject. However, there are some basic facts that are known. An embryonic steering committee was struck as a result of the 1989 Our Turn conference that Adele Rosenbloom and Dave Stewart spoke of at the beginning of this chapter. When CSDI came into being, this group asked for approximately $800,000 and received somewhat more than half that amount, $473,498 worth of ongoing operational funds, to develop an umbrella consumer and survivor organization to which all the other, smaller CSDI projects could belong. "We got big bucks," announced the OPSA newsletter in September of 1991. These, indeed, were "heady days," as Dave Stewart says.

However, trouble was not long in developing. One of the first battles was over the distinction between consumer and survivor. Initially, the organization decided that "only psychiatric survivors could vote but anyone who agrees with what we want to do is welcome to join" (*OPSAnews #4*, 1991, p. 1). Consumers, who were perceived to be less radical, did not feel welcome. CSDI, as the arm of the Ministry of Health that oversaw the terms of OPSA's funding, objected, believing that a provincial organization had to be as inclusive in its membership as possible. Some respondents were also uncomfortable with OPSA's all-survivor stance. John says, "OPSA asked me whether I was a consumer or a survivor and I refused to answer." Others agreed, feeling that the intense and emotional consumer-versus-survivor debate echoed the dehumanizing categorization of psychiatric power which members were trying to escape.

> They were polarized. Consumer was defined as someone who thinks everything is fine. You're not aware of any power imbalances and a survivor is the opposite extreme. And most people fall somewhere in between. It was just like labelling someone with mental illness. Like, what's the

difference between a psychiatric diagnosis and asking someone to fit a strict set of guidelines like OPSA was? It's all the same to me.

M. adds that a kind of gradation of misery was also part of the hurtful dynamics.

> There were a number of hierarchies that developed, all of which were dependent upon the degree to which one had suffered, ranging from how poor one's housing was to how marginalized one's employment, or unemployment, through whether one had been on the back wards or really been through the fires and been incarcerated in the Oak Ridge facility at Penetanguishene. The credentials for *real* survivor status became complex indeed.

Jennifer Chambers explains what happened next.

> We came together because of our common experience of oppression and we were all united initially and then things started to happen like someone taking on the position of leadership. And that started to echo in people the feelings towards authority—authority that they had been hurt by. On the other hand, people who were in the leadership roles felt isolated and criticized. Anyone in a prominent position who's accomplishing things tends to be the focus of attack. That's throughout society, for whatever reason. The more powerless people have been, the more likely they are to have anger against authority figures and the more likely you are to get reamed if you are one of those authority figures. But the survivor movement is probably worse than any other group I've been in. I think it's because the worse people are treated, the worse they behave to each other. We also tend not to be as afraid of each other as we are of the professionals.

Adele Rosenbloom, as a former Board member, describes what it was like to be one of OPSA's "authority figures."

> I went to an event and one guy came up to me and spit in my face. Unreal! He *spit* in my face and said, "I absolutely hate you and everything you stand for." And I had never met this person before in my life. Another women came up to me and she started screaming at me and I thought this was just insane. I was spending 20 hours a week working on

OPSA stuff at home, in addition to a full-time job and a child. It was ridiculous. There's this real problem with power and perceived power. I guess people have been put down for so long, have internalized that kind of oppression and they need a scapegoat. They need someone to strike out at and it's easier to strike out at one of their own.

Marilyn Nearing refers to this kind of infighting as cannibalism.

I see that it's about power. And the first thing you do when you grab some power is run with it. That's exactly what I did when I first got in the consumer movement. After having made some really major errors and having them reflected back to me *rather strongly*—oh, but of course for my own good. I learned. After being a survivor of sexual abuse—this type of abuse was a piece of cake.

But it was not a piece of cake for many respondents. Dave Stewart says, "It cost me to be in the middle of organizational overthrows. As politically alert and knowledgeable as I feel I am at times, being faced with these kinds of politics on a personal level threw me for a loop." M. says, "If you could only keep the power and the money separate, but you can't. As soon as somebody gets a job, it sets them apart. They have the money and the others don't."

Eventually, amidst ongoing acrimony, a failure to develop a functional Board of Directors, the public resignation of its own staff and rumours of financial irregularities, CSDI took the difficult step of recommending that the government withdraw funding.

Adele says:

We had so many opportunities. We had so much money! This wonderful organization that we'd put together from the ground up and we blew it. A lot of it was as a result of the personalities that were involved at the time but, in retrospect, I shouldn't have backed down. I should have maintained a much stronger position, but there was no support so I was in it on my own.

Hugh adds:

We fucked up. Every last person involved. Whether they kept their mouth shut or didn't or whether, like in my case, they didn't keep at it. It's the most cruel thing there is to raise people's hopes and expectations and then just not deliver, but we did that. There was just too much too fast, in view of the brain trust. Like, after the organization starves for two and a half years, the money finally comes and it comes in buckets but there were strings attached and we couldn't deal with it.

Some respondents were careful to point out that what happened at OPSA is not unique in the mental health field. Professionally run organizations have problems too. Walter Osoka says, "There have been governments that have failed. Lots of organizations have failed. As a matter of fact, there are certain professional organizations that haven't failed, but they should have." Jennifer Chambers adds:

I'm sick of hearing about the demise of OPSA. I think people's analysis of it is shallow and fragmented and lacking in compassion in all directions. It needs to be analyzed more in terms of a systems failure—Board-staff conflict is not just a consumer/survivor problem. And then you add the reality that survivors' lives are often emptier than others so that makes the strife all the more difficult. Both the Board and the staff were putting so much into it, but when there's internal dissension on top of that, it's too much for anyone to deal with.

Certainly, the dynamics within OPSA illustrate with great clarity one of the things that can go wrong in social movements. While former members have a number of explanations for the organization's failure (Shimrat, 1997), most of this study's respondents agreed that the real problem was power. Respondents and their peers seemed inexorably to recapitulate all the ills they so despised. Power as dominance became the enemy-within as members fought each other and their own leadership. The leaders, in their turn, became isolated, angry and burnt out. In specific cases, it appears that members' allegations of wrongdoing may have had some basis; in others, it was the perception, rather than the reality, that sparked attack. Simmel (in Levin, 1971) argues, like many respondents, that the extremes of oppression drive people apart rather than link them in solidarity. Prilleltensky and Gonick (1996) refer to this dynamic as internalized oppression, while Adele says simply, "It's easier to strike out at one of our own."

Janeway (1980) asks, "How often, in our time, have we not watched the dedicated efforts of some group, struggling to free themselves from oppression, and then witnessed the rebels grow obsessed by the need to hang on to the power they used for their own liberation by setting up institutions that enforce their rule over others" (p. 88). Marilyn Nearing would agree. She believes that consumers and survivors often misuse their new-found power. She says, "An elitist group of consumers can be just as detrimental as the professionals. It's not about taking power. It's about letting it flow down."

Certainly, it was my impression during the research interviews that the failure of OPSA represented a deep wound that respondents felt personally, whether they had been closely involved or not. It also seemed to represent a public shame when, as Marilyn believes, so many people were waiting and watching for just such a debacle to occur. Jennifer Chambers confirms Marilyn's feelings. "The professionals tend to make much out of any dispute among survivors." One of the major strengths of mental health professionals is that they stick together, Jennifer acknowledges. She adds, "It's a moral weakness, of course, but in terms of maintaining power, it's definitely a strength."

One of the primary tasks of effective protest, after the identification of sources of mistrust and the collective sharing of grievances, is to develop an organizational structure that will nurture and sustain leadership, rally the membership and focus their once-disparate energies (Janeway, 1980). The failure of OPSA may, in part, explain the inability of this study's respondents to see that consumers and survivors have achieved victories. Without a visible centre, a movement is in real danger of fragmenting, principally because its members, committed and individually effective though they may be, are unable to capture their successes for the development of a shared history. Instead, they experience each gain as an isolated and fragile moment that must forever be reinvented.

In conclusion

For centuries, mental patients have been deemed society's "throwaways." In the early 1990s, the Ontario government set up a fund to promote the formation of consumer and survivor organizations all over the province. In doing so, it assigned a series of complex roles to people who are stereotypically thought of as unmotivated and incompetent. The government also insisted that professionals involve consumers and survivors in all aspects of planning, developing, delivering and evaluating mental health services, elevating their endorsement to that of a legitimizing political symbol (Boudreau, 1990). In fact, consumers' and survivors' nascent political views appeared to mesh well with the government's need to restrict mental health spending through downsizing and reallocation. However, their new-found popularity, welcome though it initially may have been, did not come without a cost. The seductive call to get involved, coupled with the need to develop their own organizations, left them feeling overwhelmed and overextended. Indeed, it could be argued that flourishing self-help organizations may, in fact, be a necessary *precursor* to effective political action, principally because they allow potential movement members to develop a sense of comfort with one another in the relative safety of equal power relationships. When both demands—creating self-help organizations *and* developing a political action agenda—are visited upon a group simultaneously, neither can get the attention it deserves, placing both in jeopardy. Certainly, in this case, serious problems were evident. The development of a collective identity was interrupted by factional wrangling. And in the midst of these many difficulties, the failure of their flagship organization left consumers and survivors without a stable, provincially recognized home base to shelter them while they privately gave birth to a healthy and strong sense of solidarity.

8

Partnership

One of the signs of a vigorous government is its capacity to include those it governs in its plans. The power contract works badly when the powerful isolate themselves from their constituents and lose touch with their problems and concerns. Wise governments are attuned to any signs of escalation in dissatisfaction among the populace and judge accurately when dissent can no longer be ignored. Thus, in the early 1990s, the sudden elevation of ex-mental patients to the status of government partners could have been interpreted as a new form of power contract, one that had the potential to emphasize the views of service recipients over those of the government's traditional partners, psychiatrists and other mental health professionals. In fact, given that physicians and health care workers interpreted mental health reform as a blueprint for job loss, consumers and survivors, with their generally anti-institution and anti-psychiatry views, were among the few groups that could be counted upon to support the government's proposed changes. The invitation to participate in mental health reform, as well as many other aspects of the mental health system, placed consumers and survivors in a position of influence that was unprecedented in history, yet this study's respondents had a difficult time acknowledging this as a gain. One reason may be that consumers and survivors appear to talk about *how* the mental health system operates while government policy is much more focused on *what* and *how much*—a qualitative versus a quantitative agenda that signals a potential collision of intentions.

The threat and the promise of partnership

The threat of the partnership agenda for consumers and survivors was, of course, that it was a sham, simply a tactic to effect unpopular cost-cutting in the mental health system by shutting institutions and reallocating some jobs to cheaper community settings while simultaneously duping them into endorsing the same sorts of power dynamics of which they so vociferously complain. In short, the new and improved mental health system will be restructured and cut back, rendering it even less capable of providing the help it promises. Janeway (1980) would contend that this sort of outcome is highly likely as the maintenance of the status quo is supported through the natural inertia of the power contract. In fact, when change can no longer be avoided, the typical scenario is for established powers to admit into their midst, but not honestly welcome, a few representatives from the marginalized group in question (Goldberg, 1991). Janeway argues that these "invaders" can try and fit in all they please, but they will never qualify as bona fide members of the universe of obligation because the powerful retain exclusive rights over the definition of what is and is not "normal." An additional threat of the partnership agenda was that it might siphon off the louder, more effective advocates within the consumer and survivor movement with the seductive but hollow offer of membership in the inner circle of power, effectively robbing the movement of its leaders while at the same time putting them to work as pied pipers leading their trusting peers into a willing acceptance of their own oppression.

The promise of partnership was its potential to elevate what Foucault (1994b) calls subjugated knowledge (the everyday experiences and ideas of consumers and survivors) to a valued position which is typically occupied by formally produced and sanctioned academic and professional knowledge. For example, my work demonstrates that respondents have unique, first-hand knowledge of the mental health system which is often contrary to the professional view. They say that the system and the professionals it employs miss the point. At best, it does nothing at all, and, at worst, its misguided intentions (good or otherwise) add to their problems. When respondents asked for help, they expected the experts to provide meaningful, useful and timely assistance because that's what they're paid to do. However, they were "sadly mistaken." Janeway argues that power contracts which fail, do so because the views of the less powerful portion of the equation have been ignored. The more opportunities there are for dialogue and interaction between the powerful and the powerless, the greater the possibility of meaningful influence (Giddens, as quoted in Gadacz, 1994). Thus, the participation of consumers and survivors in all manner of activities related to the management of the mental health system held the promise of a more functional power contract, one where both academic and experiential knowledge could be respected, producing a mental health system that works.

The problems with partnership

Judi Chamberlin (1978) warns against the invasion of even well-meaning professionals into self-help organizations because they tend to influence disproportionately the goals and objectives of the membership, often diverting energy away from a liberation agenda.

Vigorous, well-established self-help organizations are one of the wellsprings from which political activism can flow. However, in the previous chapter, respondents concluded that the twin demands of founding self-help organizations while, at the same time, responding to an extensive call for partnership left them feeling overtaxed, weary and ineffective. Hugh Tapping believes that, while self-help has always been part of ex-mental patients' agenda, partnership was something new, and it didn't come from among consumers and survivors.

> I've been in and out of the movement since 1960—before it was even called a "movement"—and this sort of thing never came up. It's a government initiative to which we are responding. There has been a *complete break* between our traditional focus and what's happening now. This whole

participation thing—it sounds great but it's not something that was initiated by us. It was something those deep-thinking government policy people wanted.

However, Pat Capponi, an extremely high-profile psychiatric survivor activist, endorsed participation and, in 1989, received funding to run a leadership facilitation program. While the goal of the program was to identify and develop competent and knowledgeable leaders within the consumer and survivor movement, the clear, underlying message of the curriculum was optimism. Participation was valuable, if enough consumers and survivors could be found and trained in the foreign intricacies of board and committee etiquette. Capponi also argued for the efficacy of a more polite, co-operative approach to advocacy. While identifying the power of anger, she nonetheless taught her participants-in-the-making that an overt display of anger could be counter-productive because "the job is to reach people," and if anger gets in the way of this primary agenda then "you have failed to do your job" (Church with Capponi, 1991, p. 13).

Capponi's efforts suggest that she may well have been aware of what this study's respondents noticed—it is only a certain type of consumer or survivor who receives an invitation to participate. M. agrees:

> People tend to listen more readily to someone who looks like them. If, however, I was a little less well dressed, a little less articulate, if I hadn't adopted the social graces, if I was really angry and a shit disturber . . . it's a partnership as long as we are willing to come on the terms of the professionals.

Another respondent says that, because only a certain kind of consumer is considered "appropriate," it's always the same people who show up at the meetings.

> I'm as bad as the next person. I go to all these meetings whenever they ask me and I lay awake at night and think should I opt out of the process or should I not? Then I get there and I'm under attack by the various factions present. Like all the shit that goes with it. And you get to the table and it's always the same people. I've said everything I've

had to say and everybody knows my position. It's not like I'm vague or shy. Why don't they ask somebody else? I'm in a fairly privileged position. I have lots to eat. I went to university and it's a long time since I was in the system.

While it appears to respondents that the middle class and well educated among them are the preferred partners, even these so-called "appropriate" individuals report that their opinions are often discounted by mental health professionals and family members, causing them to feel "seen" for the purpose of recruitment and "unseen" when they try to speak out. One of the common charges they hear is, "You don't speak for the people who are really sick." This is a statement that raises hackles. Susan Marshall says:

> I got that sort of thing from a really prominent family activist—right out of her mouth. And we stood up to her as a group and said, "We don't really think it's necessary, but if you want, we can bring all our medical documentation and you can read for yourself about our psychotic experiences. We can certainly prove how 'ill' we've been." That shut her down.

Patrick Brown says:

> I'm not obligated to prove that to anybody. I know what it's like to be psychotic. I know what it is to be depressed. I also know what it is to be manic. I know what it is to experience side effects from medication. Whatever you can say about mental illness, I've been there.

Marilyn Nearing adds:

> I get that all the time, especially when dealing with the family groups. They say, "You were capable and functioning before you got ill, but my son will never be able to do that. He'll always need me to protect him and take care of him." Meanwhile we have five people in our group who have been diagnosed with schizophrenia and who have gotten their university degrees. I mean, *forgive me!* With the right support, their son might get there too. I think they've forgotten that we're crazy, not stupid.

These sorts of challenges to consumer and survivor advocacy require allegiance to a somewhat circular argument that begins with the belief that people who are deemed mentally ill are incapable of speaking on their own behalf. By this logic, people who *do* speak out can't have been mentally ill and, consequently, have nothing of value to say about those who are "really sick." This argument also requires an understanding of mental illness as a static, immutable state which, once entered, cannot be exited. Perhaps most telling of all is the demonstration of the "fundamentally incompatible discourses" between consumers, survivors and families (Boudreau & Lambert, 1993b, p. 80). Both claim a portion of the truth without a clear path to reconciliation between their opposing views. While Carling (1995) suggests that families are most effective when they stick to their own issues rather than trying to speak on behalf of others, in practice, who speaks for whom can become a muddled and emotional bone of contention.

Family challenges to consumers' and survivors' right to represent their peers lead directly to the question of who among them hasn't been invited to become the government's partners. Obviously, answers must be speculative in nature as it's impossible to know for sure who isn't present, but there are some hints. First, in the previous chapter, John remarked on the many, many ex-mental patients who are so poor that they are completely occupied by their daily search for the very basics of life: food and shelter. He feels that it's this group that gives the true meaning to the term survivor because, for them, surviving is a full-time job, leaving neither the time nor the energy for political activism. In addition, there are the many patients who remain in institutions and, although there is an effort to involve them in some level of partnership, Jennifer Chambers believes that they're afraid to speak out because they are so completely dependent on the system that they can't take the risk. On the other hand, perhaps they are satisfied with living in the institution and have little negative to say. Next, there is a group of patients and ex-patients who remain persistently psychotic and, whether in an institution or on the street, can no longer be reached, no matter what the intention. Finally, there is presumably a group of former patients that has left the system entirely. There is no real way of knowing whether they got the services they wanted and, as a consequence, represent a pool of satisfied customers who might provide a balancing perspective to consumer and survivor critiques. Alternatively, they may be people who just got out, vowing never to place themselves in the hands of professionals again. Either way, they are unavailable for recruitment as partners and their views remain a mystery.

The discussion of who's not present aside, the process of participation for the consumers and survivors who are able or willing to respond to the call for partnership has meant that they are becoming more familiar with the management and administrative workings of the mental health system. Respondents report that they are surprised at what they see. Marilyn Nearing says:

> I'm appalled at some of these professional groups. They blatantly admit that they always broke the rules and now that there are even tougher ones—I'm speaking of a housing program in this case—they are now required to have rental agreements with the residents so they make them so complex that no one can understand them and then they tell the residents, who have no resources and no money, to get a lawyer if they don't like it. Because the new rules are a pain in the ass for them, they are determined to make them a pain for consumers too.

She goes on to say:

> I've seen the staff of a psychiatric hospital just whip patients into a frenzy over this mental health reform thing. They've told them that, with shortages and cutbacks, they are likely to be out on the street next week—discharged from the only home some of them have ever known. They create a dependency and then they take that dependency and they beat the patients over the head with it, using it as a weapon to get their own needs met.

These sorts of incidents are a demonstration of resistance tactics—unadmirable though they may be—on the part of rather frightened mental health professionals. Whether they are responding to mental health reform in general, the presence of consumers and survivors in particular, or both, is unclear but these incidents represent evidence of a challenge to the status quo. In addition, such insight, if used to advantage, could become grist for the advocacy mill. However, respondents seemed not to interpret these events as indicative of the vulnerability of their "enemy," but instead see them as further evidence that the powerful are prone to betraying their trust.

The personal costs

Respondents pointed out that the partnership agenda increased the level of complexity in their relationships with professionals and this in itself became a stressor. For example, consumers and survivors are expected to debate hot topics with admitting psychiatrists who sit next to them at Ministry task forces, but who have in the past, or may in the future, commit them for involuntary treatment. I have personally experienced finishing an intense therapy session with a client in the morning only to meet the same person an hour or two later in the role of activist at a committee meeting where neither of us knew the other had been invited. These are complicated relationships to negotiate for everyone involved, compromising both the goals of respectful clinical treatment and balanced planning exercises. They also point to the presence of new and unpredictable undulations in the traditional power relations between professionals and patients, with both groups trying their best to find their balance as they navigate turbulent and uncharted waters.

Respondents also identified other personal costs which they said they were just beginning to recognize. For example, Angela Browne, writing in *OPSAnews* #7 (1992), points out that most consumers and psychiatric survivors live in poverty even though some of them are educated, articulate and in other ways indistinguishable from their mental health professional partners. Mary describes the effect this discrepancy in economic status had on her.

> We had a committee that worked well together—well, we seemed to be equals. At the end of our work, we had a celebration but when I went to the place for the party, I felt really uncomfortable. I couldn't have afforded even *one* of the pieces of the furniture in the room. I was just totally overwhelmed by the whole experience and the professionals just couldn't understand the difference. I guess the

thing was that they denied that it had such an impact on me. All I ask is just acknowledge that it has an effect and then I can stay in there and work, but don't pretend it doesn't matter.

Another cost respondents identified was the level of energy required to keep going, day after day, when they felt there were no obvious, or at least satisfactory, results to lift their spirits. Hugh says, "For three years I've worked from within the system to bring about some change but I haven't gotten anywhere." Donna adds, " One little lesson I've learned is I don't like this. I don't like the responsibility I feel to keep on shoving." Hugh goes on to explain more fully:

> When we're talking about consumers and survivors, we are talking about the walking wounded. This participation thing—well, there are some pretty heavy demands made on us and we're people who, by definition, have fewer social and emotional supports, like a lack of confidence in our ability to carry this thing forward because we don't have a 10-year career under our belt and so on. This is a heavy demand coupled with light resources and I'm not just talking about money, I'm talking about a family to go home to, having kids. Kids can keep you going. A lot of us don't have that. Therefore, expect some casualties among us. Plain and simple.

Jennifer Chambers says:

> All of it has made me more cynical about people than I have ever been before in my life. I've become more aware of what people will do to protect their own interests and that's certainly not been pleasant. I'd say that I like people less than I did before. That's hard. And you hardly ever have pleasant, caring situations when you're doing advocacy—that's another hard part. The easy part is I get to at least say how I see it, even if no one is listening.

These sorts of personal costs point to the price of advocacy when conducted in isolation. Each speaker soldiers on, but without the comfort of a home base to which he or she can return, bringing tales of victory, small and large, for celebration and preservation in group mythology. As a result, successes are lost and life as a political activist truly becomes a Sisyphean struggle.

Feeling used

Some respondents said that they have the distinct feeling that they are being used, co-opted in the language of social movements (Goldberg, 1991). Hugh Tapping says, "There are professionals out there who talk about listening to us survivors, but they only do that to get funding." Marilyn Nearing adds:

> I've seen a lot of professionals cultivating their own little group of consumers as a sort of advertising corps because they've gotten the message through mental health reform that they have to have consumers participating in their agencies and programs. They've gotten the message but they haven't gotten the *meaning*. Among ourselves we often say, "Why don't they just cut the crap?" We can tell the difference between a professional who means it and one who's just using the language.

In fact, M. believes that many consumers and survivors have a special vulnerability to the invitations they received from mental health professionals and government bureaucrats. She says, "For many of us, it's the first time anyone has ever paid attention to us." Marilyn Nearing says:

> One of the mistakes I made was that I thought I had "made it." I thought I had become a successful consumer when I found that I fit in and was accepted by the professionals. And then I realized that they weren't listening to me. It took a different degree of wellness for me to see that, but now I take great joy in being more controversial and not leaving everyone feeling cushy.

Jennifer Chambers:

> Consumer/survivor participation has been co-opted because people are getting paid to participate. Sometimes people settle for just being allowed to be there. For example, we have someone who's on a lot of hospital committees and he says, "I don't want them to know my real point of view because it's my job to be on these committees. If the administration gets angry at me, I'll be out of a job." There's never a recognition that he's there to represent what consumer/survivors want. On the other hand, people

need money. Everyone else present is paid. We should be paid too, but there should be some way of protecting us from losing our positions and the money if we take a strong oppositional stand.

This last comment points out an important change in the mechanics of consumer and survivor participation that has developed over time. During the optimistic consultation process that spawned the Graham Report (Graham, 1988), consumers and survivors reported that they "had absolutely nothing to lose and everything to gain" by participating loudly and vociferously in meetings (Church, 1993, p. 218). The reason given for this assertion was that they had no jobs to protect, unlike their more cautious bureaucratic and mental health professional adversaries and, as a result, felt no obligation to contain their emotions or edit their remarks. However, today, in recognition of the fact that it costs money to attend meetings, it has become common practice to compensate consumer and survivor participants with honoraria that can range from bus tickets to $10 or $20 per meeting. For people who typically live in poverty, $20 is an important sum. It can also be doubled, tripled or quadrupled monthly, depending on the number of meetings one has been invited to attend. In addition, because it is officially defined as an "honorarium," it constitutes an anomaly that slides by a particularly rigid social assistance rule whereby recipients must report any money earned during the month so that an equal amount may be deducted from their cheques. These factors have combined to place consumers and survivors in a position where now they, too, have something to lose.

In a more general discussion of participation, many respondents said that they didn't know exactly what was going on with all these meetings, but, whatever it was, the one thing it wasn't was partnership. Sue Goodwin says:

They have their cars and their jobs and that's never, and I mean, NEVER going to be my life. This isn't going to work until they walk through my life for a few weeks and see what it's like. I could offer some "input," as they call it, on *that* subject.

John adds:

> The government still has all the resources and we're iso-
> lated without much information at all so I don't see how
> you can call it a partnership.

Marg Oswin:

> I don't think such a thing is possible until we're regarded
> as experts in our own right.

M.:

> The Minister of Health doesn't have any idea what a part-
> nership means. I hold out some hope for one or two of the
> bureaucrats who are further down the echelon. They seem
> to have good intentions. And some professionals mean it.
> Others believe in it only if they can maintain control.

These statements assume a particular definition of partnership based on the idea that it can exist only among equals
or near equals. However, it appears that, at the time, the government assumed no such thing, although it might be criticized for using the rhetoric of partnership to describe what
was, in essence, a power contract. Janeway (1980) believes that
fears of being used may be groundless if the powerful have been
persuaded to use a movement's ideas, thereby refreshing and
invigorating the power contract with at least the promise of
improved functioning. However, this perspective assumes
merely a one-way dialogue between social movements and the
dominant powers. Movements, even in their nascent form, must
be viewed both as a cause of change—the government has to
react to their presence—and an effect—the movement must reform and adapt itself to the changes made by the those in
power (Giddens, as cited in Gadacz, 1994). In the situation
under study, respondents clearly feel that it is *they* who are
doing all the adapting while the expected governmental
changes are not forthcoming. Respondents conclude that it is
impossible to have a partnership when the power of one part of
the equation so vastly overwhelms that of the other. There is
validity to this perspective, as the reality is that, in most
instances, the government retains an inordinate level of control
in the lives of its consumer and survivor partners. For example,

it issues the social assistance cheques that most depend upon. It funds the housing in which they live. It employs their counsellors, therapists and case managers. It formulates the laws that call for a suspension of their civil rights under certain conditions. It runs the psychiatric institutions and hospitals that can hold them against their will. It even funds their own self-help and advocacy groups. Given that our society's most common experience of power is dominance, it is perhaps predictable that consumers and survivors distrusted the apparent good intentions of the partnership agenda. Mental health professionals, in their turn, seemed equally mistrustful of mental health reform and consumer and survivor involvement, indicating that the idea of partnership may be casting its seeds on stony ground.

If it's not partnership, what is it?

When respondents so clearly rejected the term partnership to describe their relationship with government, I substituted "activism" as a way of talking about their activities. However, it is a word with a rather distant, even esoteric meaning that was never used spontaneously by respondents themselves. Nevertheless, something about the word struck a chord. Paul Reeve grounded the concept with a clearer definition. He says:

> To be active means to grow. It means to strengthen. It means supporting myself and others in their journey. It is really important for me to speak from the heart around issues of healing and recovery in mental health, mental illness, whatever words you want to use. It's speaking out. It's asking the system and ourselves to respect and honour one another.

Paul's definition agrees with those that are more formally produced. Hooks (1989) defines politicization as, first, recognizing the personal experience of exploitation and, second, as "understanding the particular structure of domination that has caused it" (p. 107), while Prilleltensky and Gonick (1996) speak of empowerment as "the power to give self and others an equal voice in society" (p. 13). Activism, however, is the aspect of politicization that demands that people do something about their situation.

The principal outlet for most respondents' activism has been the occasions when they represent their fellow consumers and survivors on boards, committees and task forces. During these times, they say, as Paul does, that it is their mission to "speak from the heart" and tell the truth. However, there were other dimensions to their political activism that respondents wished understood.

Jennifer Reid explains:

> The movement has given me a sense of belonging. I'm part Native, part black and I'm adopted. There are no roots for me. The psychiatric survivor movement didn't take me as a lesbian, a radical or a feminist. They took me as a survivor—a survivor who told the truth and who had something to say.

Marg Oswin says:

> It's given me my identity. It gives me a sense of who I am, where I've been. I'm more than just a statement of facts. I'm a real, three-dimensional person. It gives me my strength and power. When I'm speaking with survivors about what we need from each other, it takes a load off my shoulders because I can share with them on a level that I can't share with anybody else. When I'm speaking to people who are not survivors and I'm pounding my head on the wall—*again*, I think, are they just not hearing me? What am I doing here? Many times, I just want to say, well, I've done everything I can so it's time to move on, but I find that I see more suffering and I respond.

Marilyn Nearing adds:

> It gives me the most excitement I've had in my life. I no longer wake up in the morning and think, why on God's earth was I born? It gives me my purpose in life. It gives me great satisfaction.

Patrick Brown:

> I think one of the good things is that when you do a deed and can look back and see that it's been implemented, that gives you a good feeling. It's also good to hear nice com-

ments from people. That boosts my ego and my self-esteem. It gives me self-fulfilment. It also gives me confirmation that, hey, I'm not such a bad guy after all.

Although respondents feel that, while it has not been a partnership that has developed, whatever *is* going on has not been a total loss. Dave Stewart says that he's learned a lot.

> It's helped me deal positively with a lot of anger. It has also focused me. It's taught me that I can't be the wild-eyed radical that I used to be. I still tend to get more publicly angry than I should and probably alienate people, but I have tried, without selling out, to understand other points of view and I've also tried to figure out ways to get my own point of view across so that people will hear me. I have also come to appreciate that I'm not going to get everybody sold. I can't believe myself sometimes when I become a bit defensive on behalf of the "establishment." I'm not defending them as much as trying to point out that there are two sides to this, folks. I mean I never thought I'd be doing that.

Susan Marshall adds that she's found a job through her activism and it's extremely important to her.

> My past history was that I would get a job, do well for a few months and then start the cycle of overwork and then get ill and then I'd either quit or I'd get fired, one of the two. So when I took this job, a similar thing happened. Within a year, I was down again, but luckily I was able to pull out of it. AND I still had the job. I didn't have to hide the reason that I was off work. It freed me, I mean, the job itself, but it's more the whole movement really. It freed me to be open and honest in my life. It's made me financially independent, which is really important to me—not dependent on the system or a husband.

She goes on to say:

> And the people I've met—it's just fantastic. I can cross the province and know survivors everywhere. Even meeting people who work for the government—the so-called bureaucrats that I had a real contempt for before. I've worked with some of them who just give and give and give. It's fantastic when you meet people who, at least to my knowledge, aren't survivors, yet they give so much.

Marilyn Nearing agrees. She says:

> There are two professionals in our area that I met through
> my participation as a consumer in the mental health sys-
> tem and I'll tell you, when you get a professional who has a
> real belief system based on values, when they don't feed
> into the language of the system or act out of political expe-
> diency, they can do so much for us.

It appears, then, that when the personal becomes political,
it is in the personal portion of the equation where consumers
and survivors see and appreciate gains. It is also in this micro-
domain that professionals emerge as whole human beings
instead of the stereotypes described in chapter 6. Nevertheless,
respondents remained clear that even like-minded professionals
are not a part of their movement. Mary explains:

> It's hard for us to recognize that we have allies—to trust
> that these people, although they have professional status,
> are willing to work with us. The reality is, though, we can-
> not ignore the differences.

Gadacz (1994) says that whenever professionals and consumers
interact, whether in direct service situations or at the level of
planning and managing, their relationship is a dialectical one,
"characterized by both unity and the struggle of opposites"
(p. 76). They converge in their desire to have a system that
works, but diverge on the subject of control. Paul Reeve states:

> As far as I can see, consumers and survivors want auton-
> omy and respect. Autonomy being freedom of choice and
> the support to make that choice and respect being an
> understanding that I am both worthy and capable. I don't
> think we have an agreement that professionals share these
> values. They also need to be more human. They need to be
> able to say that they don't know it all. They need to stop
> being a "treatment" or a "philosophy" and just be human.

Naming themselves as "activists" appears to have more appeal
than "partners" because it captures more accurately the nature
of their critique, while, at the same time, acknowledges their
fighting spirit. Activists are independent, honourable and committed. They don't give in and they don't sell out. They are
demonstrably separate from the powers they assail. They are the

modern-day version of warriors, lonely, isolated and rather dispirited as it has been demonstrated, but nonetheless warriors who have discovered their purpose and found their place in the world.

Will mental health reform work?

The publication of the Graham Report represented a period of intense optimism for the consumers and survivors who were present during the consultations that led up to its release. Marg Oswin says, "Those were the glory days when we thought anything was possible." Pat Capponi (1992a) agrees. "Everywhere we went ex-patients stood up and described how hopeless their lives had become thanks to poverty, isolation and horrible housing. It was a strong message: Do something!" (p. 208). However, *Putting People First* made respondents worried. While, as Paul Reeve says, it seems to have been intended as an endorsement of motherhood, apple pie and the flag, all rolled into one, a closer reading exposed some disturbing problems. John explains:

> *Putting People First* was produced by some people at the Ministry offering their own views about what was needed. I still don't know who wrote it. How did they come up with those service priorities?

Patrick Brown says:

> In my opinion, they should have done some research to see if any of this will work because nobody knows. The idea might sound good, but who knows? It might also be destructive.

Marnie Shepherd asks, in exasperation:

> When are they ever going to stop writing papers and actually do something? Let's stop talking about it and get started.

In fact, respondents felt that the only concrete outcome of the seemingly never-ending planning process, spawned by the Graham Report and reinforced by *Putting People First*, was the growing sense that the call to partnership had, in fact, pitted consumers and survivors against psychiatrists and the unions that represent hospital workers. Donna says:

The people who are expected to implement mental health reform are the very people who are threatened with job loss and will do everything they can to fight against change. The government, their boss, has come out with this plan and they have to *act* as if they're behind it, but they're really going to sabotage it and there can be no doubt about it.

Marilyn Nearing adds:

Coming on too strong with this sort of policy can cause a backlash. Mental health professionals are really afraid of losing their jobs. It's just pitted two vulnerable groups— labour and the mentally ill—against one another, although there are a whole lot of reasons to believe that consumers and survivors are more vulnerable than the labour force.

Mary:

The major issues are those of the unionized workers, job loss and retraining. I don't see our issues—poverty, for example—coming first at all. It's all about jobs. We stay poor and they benefit from our despair.

Sue Goodwin concludes:

Honest to God, my only hope is that survivors will be able to grab a chunk of the money and keep making our voices heard.

The idea that the consumer and survivor movement, with its typically anti-institution stance, may be providing government with a utilitarian logic that will serve as a saleable argument for downsizing or closing expensive psychiatric hospitals was not at all far-fetched, as time has shown. The above comments also emphasize respondents' earlier fears that they may become targets for retaliation. The fact that consumer and survivor activism has created an environment where mental health professionals have become afraid could be seen as evidence of a victory, but it is one that respondents feel has a dangerous double edge. Government bureaucrats seemingly welcome them with open arms at the planning table, but they won't be present on the admitting ward to provide protection should their former "partner" suffer a breakdown and require hospitalization. Indeed, consumers' and survivors' stories are full of accounts of the small, cruel abuses that can take place on a psychiatric ward, regardless of regulatory policies and procedures. They know that all the rules in the world won't protect them if no one is looking.

Such fears are all the more powerful because they encourage disconnection from a calm, rational assessment of probability. While consumer and survivor activists may, indeed, be well known if they reside in small towns or in rural areas, only the most prominent activists have any public profile at all in large urban centres. It is entirely likely that harried hospital admitting staff and overworked ward professionals would have no idea of the political activism of their patients. However, the individual activists would know, and the experience of having re-entered their former powerless patient role would be all the more humiliating because of the heightened contrast between it and the new status conferred by political activity.

An additional source of concern for consumers and survivors is the fact that plans developed at a bureaucratic level are a long, long way from the realities of the direct service interface between professional and patient—arguably the most salient power contract in the entire mental health system. When the present study began, mental health reform planning had already been underway for six years, and respondents were clear that they were beginning to lose faith that the hundreds of documents it had produced would ever be translated into real, observable change.

Donna:

> We've never redistributed the money in any real way like the politicians promised so there's nothing that's been added to the community. So, we're set up for failure just like in the '70s. We're going to wind up with all the crazies on the street with none of the supports, no housing, no money and they'll be disruptive, they'll be visible, and there will be a big social outcry and then they'll get re-incarcerated in the institutions all over again.

Jane Pritchard:

> They're lying through their teeth and they know it. They don't have the money to do what it is that they said they would and they don't tell people that.

Mary:

> I know they used the words, "putting people first," but the power imbalances haven't been addressed so I don't see a whole lot changing.

While some respondents feel that *Putting People First* might possibly have been based on good intentions, they believed it would become derailed during implementation discussions. One reason may be that plans have tended to focus mostly on targets such as bed reductions and the problems associated with the redeployment of unionized staff to community-based jobs. Respondents believe that their concerns, which concentrate on how the system functions rather than how much it costs, have been lost, while, at the same time, some feel that the only observable result of so-called partnership is to have pitted consumers and survivors against powerful unions who are, indeed, facing a serious threat. Respondents conclude that mental health reform cannot work if the fundamental qualitative issue—how power is used—is not addressed, first, in the mental health system as a whole and, second, in its key direct service functions. Gadacz (1994) states that professionals and consumers have yet to agree on a change in the nature of this extremely important power contract. In this case, consumers and survivors say, "We want autonomy and respect." However, there appears to be no real evidence that professionals have altered their traditional stance which says, "We are the experts and we know best." Finally, adding to the anxiety and frustration, action of any sort was exceedingly slow in coming. In the process, endless planning fuelled everyone's fears. Consumers and survivors feared retaliation, psychiatrists feared a loss of power, other professionals feared for their jobs, unions feared the general anti-labour tenor that is evident in some of the plans, families feared an erosion of services and the community mental health sector feared that the promised program enhancements would never arrive.

In such an atmosphere of instability, the professional position is a shaky one. Their power is eroding. Many of the institutions that have employed them are slated for closing, and the unions that have protected their jobs are under attack (Armstrong & Armstrong, 1996). However, mental health care is an activity where the primary resource is people. *Putting People First* (1993) is virtually silent on the issue of its own impact on the people who work in the mental health system. Important employee support measures such as education and training, well-thought-out systems for reallocation to community jobs and a strategy to address remuneration differentials are absent. It is no great leap of logic to presume that unhappy, downtrodden and threatened workers are likely to produce an even poorer standard of care than the supposed deficiencies that sparked reform in the first place. Throughout the eternal and, it must be noted, enormously expensive planning exercise that was the only tangible product arising out of the early part of mental health reform, professionals found themselves side by side with consumers and survivors, creating policies that may well herald the demise of their own institutions, hospitals and agencies— manufacturing a do-it-yourself hangman's kit—as survivor activist Colin Young is rumoured to have said in a show of sympathetic black humour. While the consumer and survivor voice has been an important and virtually absent ingredient in mental health discourse, pitting it against the interests of medicine and labour can hardly improve quality of care in either the short or the long term. In short, mental health professionals seem to have joined the ranks of the disempowered, and they appear to have no immediate way out of their dilemma. Government can take the ideological high ground and argue that it is merely acting as a responsible representative of its taxpayers' concerns. In the same vein, consumers and survivors can comfort themselves that they are the champions of a forgotten but essential group that requires vigorous representation no matter whose feelings get hurt. And finally, family members take the entirely sympathetic stance that it's their loved ones they are fighting for. But mental health professionals, the people relied on to provide the improved care that mental health reform is designing, are embattled on all sides. Consumers, survivors and often family members view them with contempt, while their own employers are threatening them with job loss. In the midst of these dynamics, professionals seem to have been assigned the role of villain. Those who take an advocacy stance on behalf of their patients or clients are seen as using them to advance their own interests while, if they stand up for their own rights as employees, they are viewed as selfish turf-protectors. While the power relations in the mental health system could be said to have shifted, it would appear that from the professional perspective, as well as from the viewpoint of consumers and survivors, mental health reform isn't working at all.

In conclusion

For respondents, the hope associated with the call to partnership early in the reform process was its potential to affect qualitatively the nature of the mental health power contract on both micro and macro levels. Their presence on literally hundreds of Boards of Directors, committees, planning groups and task forces certainly represents a change, but they report that many of the same aspects of the dominant power relationship they experienced while patients or clients in direct service settings are reproduced in the macro areas of system planning and management. They feel they are selected because of their middle-class backgrounds and education, yet they are attacked because they "don't speak for really sick people." Some say that, despite the initial welcoming rhetoric, their ideas were ignored. Many feel used, recruited merely as a counterweight to the power of psychiatrists and unions who are threatened by the government's emphasis on fiscal restraint. In the midst of the turmoil everyone is afraid, and the promise of a reformed, invigorated and functioning mental health system appears to be receding. In fact, respondents, psychiatrists (OPDPS, 1994) and unions (OPSEU, 1991, 1994) seem to be reaching similar conclusions. Mental health reform, as articulated in *Putting People First*, is viewed as an administrative document, concerned mainly with system management and cost-effectiveness, relegating important qualitative concerns such as *how* services are delivered to a secondary status. A significant missing piece, however, is a solid consumer and survivor advocacy position offered in a strong, clear voice. While there are hints that they embrace a form of liberation ideology, *exactly* what they believe in as a collectivity may be a question that consumers and survivors themselves have yet to answer.

9

What do consumers and survivors believe in?

Consumers and psychiatric survivors appear to want qualitative changes in the mental health system—changes that have to do with a fundamental alteration in the nature of both the macro-level power contract (how the entire mental health system operates) and the micro-level power contract (how professionals help their patients and clients)—but what, specifically, does that mean? One of the tasks of a viable social movement is to create a creed or an ideology which functions as its *cri de coeur*. Creeds are expressed in a variety of ways. Sometimes they are contained in lengthy mission statements or manifestos. At other times they are reduced to catchy slogans or songs, but, no matter what their form, their function is to rally the membership so that they are marching under the same banner. The power of a creed lies in its ability to connect members' emotional commitment to a rational, well-thought-out agenda for change. If a rising sense of uneasiness has made the powerful restless and they have come to call, asking "What do you want?" movements benefit if they are ready with a clear answer. For example, the women's movement has rallied around the slogan, "The personal is political." As a creed, it is somewhat curious in that, on one hand, it uses powerful words that denote strength of purpose while, on the other, it requires a considerable amount of thought and effort to figure out exactly what it means. Nevertheless, it has served as a legitimizing symbol for feminists and, many years after its invention, continues to colour their personal, academic, business and political lives. In a second example, the public has come to understand that, while the physically disabled may want many things, they *demand* accessibility. They have been hugely successful in pressuring governments, businesses and transportation companies into making costly structural alterations so that people in wheelchairs and the blind can navigate the able-bodied world as independently as possible.

So far, the current expression of the consumer and survivor movement appears not to have been able to settle upon such a clearly defined agenda for change. Hugh Tapping states that the government's partnership agenda constituted a complete break from what an earlier version of the movement had in mind. This previous ideology seemed to centre around Chamberlin's 1978 call for self-help and survivor-run alternative services. Today, with consumers and survivors participating in unprecedented numbers in a wide variety of activities related to all aspects of the mental health system, the development of a coherent ideology has become a more complex task than when they were fewer in number and their activism went virtually unnoticed. One potential reason for their seeming lack of clarity may be that the invitation to partnership diverted them from the task of developing their own ideas for change.

Under ideal circumstances, the evolution of a movement's ideology is a difficult task, because so many things may be wrong that it's hard to sort out exactly what to concentrate on. Indeed, respondents have remarked upon the difficulty of retaining their focus when so many things need changing. Second, it is the powerful who know how things work, and consumers and survivors have had limited access to even the most basic facts and figures so that they can advocate effectively for themselves. John confirms this perception. He says, "We're isolated without much information at all." Finally, in order to create an ideology, movement members must first understand how the powerful function, and, in the light of that knowledge, develop persuasive and compelling counterarguments that address the difficult task of changing long-term, well-established and embedded traditions—a daunting task that leaves even the strongest movement members frustrated. As Marg Oswin says, "I pound my head on the wall. Is it me or is it them?"

In this chapter, I attempt to find out what it is that consumers and survivors believe in. I began with the questions, what do you think mental illness is and what do you think should be done about it? I was particularly interested in the first part of this question because how a problem is defined dictates the choice of solution. I expected respondents to offer a powerful counter-definition of mental illness rooted in first-hand experience. Who better to define a phenomenon than those who are closest to it? And what better way to found an ideology than to reappropriate the power to define one's own experience. While their answers as reported below are thoughtful, it was, in fact, the second part of the question, What did they think should be done about it? where the passion lay.

It's a chicken or egg thing

Historically, discussions around the etiology of insanity or mental illness have polarized around the age-old nature-nurture debate. Is it an inescapable biological fault expressed as a disease or is it socially created, a sane response to an insane world? Treatment responses are also split: physical remedies for the biologically based proponents and talk therapies for those who believe more in social causality (Pilgrim & Rogers, 1993). Janeway (1980) states that we seem doomed to view these sorts of complex problems in "binary terms" (p. 305). Life divides into black and white, right and wrong, yes and no, and these divisions are based on our view of power as dominance, a view that creates only two ranks within the power contract: the haves and the have nots, the powerful and the powerless, the strong and the weak. These two ranks are often cast in direct opposition to one another, win or lose, harm or be harmed.

The respondents of this study initially reported that they felt that people who call themselves psychiatric survivors typically support the nurture side of the mental illness debate (social causality), while consumers are those who embrace the nature side (biological etiology). In practical terms, respondents, although identifying politically as survivors, reported that they actually lived their lives somewhere in between these nature-nurture explanations, sometimes taking medications and "consuming" services and sometimes not, a precarious balancing act from the perspective of their typically antiprofessional stance. In fact, the question—what is mental illness?—seemed to touch places that were intimate and hard to talk about. Respondents paused for some time after I asked it, and often remarked, "That's an *interesting* question." Most answers did not come easily. Two respondents had less difficulty than others and answered with a well-thought-out, personal philosophy statement which, in Jennifer Chambers's case, seemed to be based on her experiences as a peer counsellor. Jennifer says:

> I think that what happens is that when people are hurt, they develop difficulty in thinking in those areas in which they were hurt. The natural way people heal from the hurt is to express emotion and get loving attention. If we aren't allowed that, we build up more areas in which we have difficulty thinking and that's what ends up being called mental illness. These hidden feelings finally break through and they are considered to be manic or psychotic, or you have people who are so successful at keeping themselves shut down, they're diagnosed as clinically depressed. I believe that what people refer to as delusions and psychoses are an attempt of the brain to sort out stressful events symbolically, like dreaming does when we're asleep. I think that it's possible for almost everyone who has a label of mental illness to be much better than they are, but there would need to be a lot of love and a lot of attention. It would require widespread societal change because I think changes in child-rearing techniques would be the way to start.

Donna's philosophy also seems based on her own personal experience:

This thing that we've labeled mental illness is really just sadness and discouragement. These feelings have a natural function—they're a normal response to abnormal situations. But we've got professionals to convince us that there's something wrong with feeling that way and that we need to go out and get help to help alleviate these problems. We're taught that it's not normal instead of embracing our pain and understanding that feeling sad is just as normal as feeling happy. So, we end up with a whole bunch of people saying there's something wrong with the way that we're behaving and medicalizing it so that we have diseases.

Other respondents were more tentative. Susan Marshall says:

At first I thought that there was no such thing as mental illness. It was a reaction to abuse or trauma—people's different coping mechanisms. I still think that's a large part of what happens—a really large part. But I'm starting to be open to the thought that there's something chemical that happens in the brain and respect people's beliefs on that.

Dave Stewart:

Something's wrong, that's for sure. It may come out of great trauma or there may be some biological, chemical or physiological maladjustment—I'm just very sceptical of the term mental illness. I think it has been badly abused and poorly understood.

Mary:

I guess it's the oscillation between hope and despair that all of us go through. I will never accept anyone who says it's one hundred percent biological or that it's one hundred percent non-biological. I've seen medication improve some people's lives and I've seen the devastation it creates. I think people have to develop their own understanding of their experience.

Paul Reeve concludes:

I can create all sorts of chemicals in my body due to my interactions with the world. It's a chicken or egg thing.

Some respondents felt that child abuse was at the bottom of it all. Jane Pritchard says:

> I think that so-called mental illness has to do with spirit killing and I believe that for most people it begins in early childhood. If your spirit is killed before you even get going, you don't know how to live, you don't take care of yourself and I don't mean just physically. I mean you don't learn how to nurture yourself and to have a sense of yourself. An abusive childhood causes people to develop different ways of coping that end up looking like strange behaviours which are not accepted by society. Yet, these behaviours are perfectly normal to them and are, in fact, what kept them alive, at least in body if not in spirit.

Marg Oswin:

> I was sexually abused when I was a child and that led to other things that eventually put me into the system. If indeed I was depressed, it was associated with a life event and not with a disease of the mind. If people have neuro-logical problems, you can call that an illness but *any* ill-ness is associated with the body, mind, spirit and emotions. What they call mental illness is an emotional dis-ease that is best treated with therapy, not with electric shock.

Sue Goodwin:

> It's abuse, all through your life, starting as a child. You can't be cured of abuse by drowning your mind in drugs that make you forget. You have to take responsibility for yourself, but you can only do that once you understand and are helped by talking it through. In my case, talk and talk and talk and talk.

Marnie Shepherd:

> The more consumers and survivors I meet, the more and more I think of the environmental impact. Early on in my understanding of this, I met somebody who had been sexu-ally abused. She is a twin. She was the only sister that was sexually abused by her father. She would tell stories of what he would do and how he would have card parties and bring home the men and it was just *awful*. I look at her and here she is in her late twenties and I just don't think the day's

ever going to come when she's going to think well of herself because there's never going to be an answer. Why did
he abuse her and not her twin sister? And I think it's never
going to matter how many people tell her it's not her fault,
it's never going to go away.

Finally, a few respondents felt that "what is mental illness?" wasn't a question that was worth the bother of answering. Walter Osoka says, "It's many things, loneliness, social
pressures, loss of a job or a loved one, lack of support, not fit-
ting in. Pinpointing a definition is a waste of time." Patrick
Brown, who says on one hand, "Whatever you can say about
mental illness, I've been there," nevertheless, felt stumped by
this question. He said, "It's very simple. I don't know."

In the main, respondents' definitions of mental illness
were tentative, despite the fact that they have experienced it
firsthand. One reason may be that the stigma attached to a
diagnosis of mental illness is so great that consumers and survivors simply do not wish to torture themselves further by
engaging in an internal debate about what *really* went wrong—
for fear of what they might discover. Second, and perhaps a
more compelling reason in the context of this work, is the reality that consumers and survivors have a history of relating to
one another in the binary, black-and-white terms of dominance,
with one group defined as willing participants in their own
oppression and the other as wise keepers of the political truth.
In practical terms, this split has made members of both camps
embarrassed to admit to one another that they take medication
or "consume" mental health services, and for good reason.
Those who reveal that they have a psychiatrist on whom they
rely, a program they value or a medication that has worked risk
attack for consorting with the "enemy." Defining mental illness, especially in an overt collective sense, brings them into
emotionally explosive territory where tempers flare, insults are
thrown and feelings are hurt. Under these circumstances, many
may indeed decide that, for the sake of solidarity (and their own
emotional safety), the question is best left unanswered, and in
some cases, even unconsidered.

Chamberlin (1978) states that "mental illness" is the kind
of "large" problem that taps into much bigger human issues

which are often the province of philosophers—what and where is the mind? What are emotions, thoughts and ideas, and how are they produced and acted upon? The connection between the mind and the body is, in some quarters, being rethought or, as some would say, reestablished, given the traditional emphasis in medicine on the Cartesian mind-body split. For example, epidemiologists who study the general health of whole populations, both historically and in contemporary times, argue that most of our health care policy is based on simple "repair shop" notions of health and illness—when something goes wrong, the offending body part must be isolated and then fixed or replaced (Evans, 1994). When mind and body are viewed as interrelated, and defying disentanglement, the polarized nature-nurture debate that characterizes mental health disappears, and in its place emerge viewpoints such as those offered by most of this study's respondents—mental illness is a little bit of both. Evans (1994), like the respondents, concludes, "genetic and congenital factors are not unimportant but the expression or non-expression of their effects depends on social environment" (p. 20). In fact, this author reports that the most pervasive finding in epidemiological studies of population health is that the less control people have over their lives, the more stress they are under and, as a consequence, the poorer their physical and mental health.

Gil's (1996) theoretical framework, which identifies our society as structurally violent, hypothesizes that one of the effects of initiating social violence is that it prevents large groups of society's outsiders from meeting even their basic human needs. In light of the above set of epidemiological findings, this sort of endemic violence would create a tremendous effect on health and, by extension, health care costs. In addition, in the specific case of child abuse, van der Kolk (1987; van der Kolk & Fisler, 1994) links trauma to chemical changes in the brain that affect the ability to regulate thoughts and emotions, interpreting scientifically what respondents seem to have understood intuitively—physical, emotional or sexual abuse produces permanent alterations in the functioning of the autonomic and central nervous systems. Further, it has been found that the greatest impairment is experienced by adults who were violently abused very early in life, for long periods of time, by multiple abusers, usually including a parental figure (Brown & Finkelhor, 1986; Goff et al., 1991). However, child abuse, along with domestic violence and rape, are only a few examples of the sorts of experiences that thwart human potential. Evans (1994) points to other problems such as poverty, often concomitant with poor housing, inadequate nutrition and an inability to achieve an education, as predictive of poor health. In addition, Ontario is a favoured destination of immigrants and refugees who bring with them a unique set of stressors related to lack of employment, an inability to speak either of Canada's official languages, the loss of friends and family and racism. Some are refugees who have experienced rape, torture and confinement in concentration camps or prisons. Women, children and old people appear to suffer the most (Durbin & Sondhu, 1992, p. 6). Finally, First Nations people experience at least four times the suicide rate of non-Native Ontarians, and are known to struggle with inferior housing, poverty, racism, substance abuse problems, unemployment, child abuse and violence (Graham, 1988). All of these social problems have vast implications for both physical and mental health.

Evans and Stoddart (1994) state that these sources of stress, and many others that may be rooted in idiosyncratic experience, are the kinds of things that place strain on the human organism which, in turn, leads to an experience of suffering. However, whether or not people define their discomfort as a health concern depends, first, on their expectations of what the health care system can deliver and, second, on the ready availability of services. In the case of this study, respondents reported that they struggled sometimes for long periods of time before they turned to the mental health system in hopes that the experts would "fix it." Indeed, the express purpose of medicine is to redefine patients' experiences of suffering as disease. This translation process—from dis-ease to disease, as respondent Marg Oswin calls it—is then accompanied by a treatment protocol and a prediction of outcome. It appears that it is at this point where respondents felt the system began to let them down. Help, as they defined it, was not forthcoming and, instead, many encountered either the vio-

lence of involuntary psychiatric treatment or nothing—no help
and no answers.

What needs to change?

In chapter 5, respondents discussed what they had
hoped the mental health system would deliver when they
approached it for help. Jennifer Reid says, "I believed that they
would fix things so that I would get better . . . be able to go out
into society." Patrick Brown adds:

> We need empathy. We want to hear, "Hey, you can make
> it!" If you place your confidence in people, I think you'd
> get the kind of results that would blow you away. Most sur-
> vivors don't have confidence and that's what they need.

Paul Reeve advises:

> Ask us what we need. Don't tell us. It's wonderful to give
> a person who's in pain some responsibility—support,
> too—but responsibility for choosing their own direction.
> That's empowering and is, in itself, part of the recovery
> process.

Mary:

> It's not about theories and textbooks. It's about simple
> things. Just by giving a person the time of day, we're
> telling them they are of value and that's not taught in
> school. You have to allow people to sense that you really
> believe in them and you believe in their abilities. There are
> some real, real issues and you don't have to be a consumer
> to see that they are important—like poverty and housing.
> If a person is discharged from hospital with all they own
> packed into a garbage bag—well, how stable are you going
> to be living out of a garbage bag? Like, simple, simple
> issues that need to be addressed. And isolation. I would say
> that the people in the *most* need are those who are so iso-
> lated. I was there—I was one of them. And you have to be
> patient and you have to just be there with a message of
> "Yes, I care." And it takes an extended period of time and
> it isn't about taking control of someone's life or using
> power. It's about very basic people skills and I don't think
> we concentrate at all on these things.

Jennifer Chambers:

> There need to be places where people can go—places of
> real healing, loving, supportive places where people would
> be allowed to show emotion. Almost everyone in society is
> afraid of emotion—especially mental health professionals.
> It's not cool for people to be sobbing endlessly, but that's
> what many of us need to do.

An anonymous respondent:

> People's problems are individual and that's where the fail-
> ure is. We have a system. And then we have individuals. We
> have models. And then we have individuals. A system or a
> model doesn't take into account people's differences.

Concluding the discussion, Mary adds an addendum to her
statement above:

> When I first started in this movement, I had never used the
> terms social control or oppression. Those words were just
> *so hard* to speak, but when I really began to look at what
> they meant and what function the mental health system
> has in our lives, I think we, as a society, have to ask our-
> selves, what role are we asking psychiatrists and other
> mental health professionals to play? Is it social control or
> is it health care? I think we are getting to the point where
> there are some real ethical questions we need to address,
> but people are still beating around the bush—not looking
> at the real issues and not discussing them openly.

In discussing some of the ethical questions that Mary
speaks of, respondents named a number of concerns, beginning
with the central question of involuntary treatment.
Walter Osoka:

> I don't think storing up people in institutions is the way to
> do it. How would someone with diabetes do if they were out
> on the streets without a place to go, without friends—
> where someone can put them in a room, lock it up and
> take away their basic right to say yes or no. How do you
> think they would fare?

A second ethical question for respondents is the powerful role
that pharmaceutical companies play in the system.

Sue Goodwin:

> The government always says it's too expensive to do the
> things that we want done. In fact, I think it would be
> *cheaper*. It costs billions to lock people up and drug them.
> They drug us in the institutions. They drug us in the jails.
> They can even drug us in our communities. But it's not
> cheaper in the long run. The government pays through
> OHIP bills and we pay through our hearts. Big time.

A third issue was work. *Putting People First* fails even to mention
employment, an absolutely central concern for many respondents.
  John:

> People need jobs—their own income so they can be really,
> truly independent. The way it is now, people get out of hos-
> pital and they're on social assistance. Having your own
> income means you're more likely to recover and be less
> dependent on all those community supports that they're
> talking about under mental health reform.

Walter Osoka:

> Someone once said, "It's amazing how somebody's emo-
> tional health gets better when they have some money and
> food, a roof over their heads and some friends."

Respondents also felt that the important issue of child abuse
seems to receive very little attention.
  Marilyn Nearing:

> I'm adamant that if professionals understood the abuse
> that underlies so-called mental illness, we'd have it whipped.

The global term that respondents most often used to
describe what they wanted was support, "emotional and economic support," says Marilyn Nearing. Evans (1994) states that
"a supportive environment helps us bear heavier loads without
breaking" (p. 22). Support, as defined by this study's respondents, is twofold. First, there are the intangible, emotional components associated with the kind of support offered by friends,
family and community which, ideally, include respect, empathy,
interest, love, encouragement, acceptance, guidance, understanding, patience, faith in one's capabilities, a shoulder to cry
on, a space to express difficult emotions, a listening ear, a place

to belong and a reason to live, to name some of the needs expressed by respondents. A second component of support is its more tangible economic aspect, sometimes called broader health determinants (Evans, Barer & Marmor, 1994): housing, income, decent food, safe communities, an education and a job. Of course, this list of needs is all too familiar, given that it includes exactly the same sorts of things my own former patients said that they wanted: friends, family, a home and a job. However, as professionals, I and my colleagues were unable to provide these sorts of supports and, instead, translated patients' expression of suffering into a psychiatric diagnosis which, in turn, led to things like hospitalization, medication and ECT, marginalization, poverty, unsafe and inferior housing, violence and many of the other hard realities that typify patients' lives. In fact, respondents repeatedly charge that professionals miss the point, fail to help and actually make their problems worse through the trauma of involuntary treatment and the stigma of psychiatric diagnosis.

What are consumers and survivors going to do about it?

It is Chamberlin's (1978) point of view that mental health professionals don't get it, haven't gotten it for over two centuries and aren't likely to get it in the near future. Thus, it is time for consumers and survivors to take charge of their own health. However, she warns that they have a very difficult task ahead of them, one that requires energy, commitment, faith and a lot of time. Respondents felt that they were becoming weary. Paul Reeve says:

> We don't want to end up victims in a survivor role. We need to work on our own healing, move into an empowered position ourselves. We have to understand that we don't just exist to change the mental health system.

Adele Rosenbloom:

> I'd like there to be some sort of wonderful coming together of all these different survivors groups where there's a real respect and sharing, where people listen to each other and support each other. We need to say, "OK,

> let's forget the past. Let's heal the wounds and move on and create something new."

M.:

> I'm hoping we'll come together. We haven't yet. Hopefully we'll realize that for all our differences, our goals are the same and we'll begin to work together better than we have in the past. I don't think it's anybody's fault that we don't work well together. With all the problems we've had, it's a miracle that anybody's working at all.

Despite very similar goals that could have formed the basis of an ideology, many respondents felt isolated, demoralized and battle fatigued—"victims in a survivor role." Mary says, "I think what has happened with all this participation business, and the funding opportunities that went with it, is that we've actually slowed down our development—or stopped it—stopped what would have been a grass-roots movement."

Throughout the entire research project, many respondents prefaced their remarks about mental health professionals and government bureaucrats with the statement, "I think their intentions were good," but McKnight (1994) calls this the most dangerous explanation there is. He insists that if people look beneath the rhetoric of "doing good," they will see that a justification of good intention is no guarantee whatsoever that a positive outcome will result. Certainly, from the perspective of the theoretical context of this work, the guise of "doing good" is the essential companion to a power contract based on dominance. As respondents have demonstrated, dominance can be experienced in many forms—from the overt coercion of involuntary treatment, easily recognized for what it is, to the much more subtle tactic of a suspect call to partnership based on the invisible practices of hegemonic dominance. This latter form of power contract is, by definition, much more difficult to identify and navigate. However, it has also presented consumers and survivors with opportunities for an unprecedented level of influence along with the difficulties. Relative to the "old days," consumers and survivors now have a substantial resource base which, although it has netted them their own self-help and economic development organizations, has brought with it its own stresses and strains. In the face of these good news/bad news contradictions, respondents feel burned out and frustrated, but they're also energized, committed and, in some cases, fighting mad. However, a still-missing ingredient in their campaign for change is a clear ideology which is critical for the safe navigation among and between the competing claims of their fellow "stakeholders."

Disability rights

The respondents of this study have emphasized the need for a change in the power contract—a long-term, societally based and fundamental change that challenges our beliefs from the micro perspective of how we raise our children to the macro concern of how we provide mental health care. One of the primary tactics for creating change, which could have been part of a fledgling ideology but one which was *not* mentioned in any significant way by respondents, is an emphasis on civil rights. Rights are protections, usually enshrined in law, which are accorded the powerless so that they are insulated against accidental or intentional abuse perpetrated within the confines of the power contract. Advocacy based solely on a rights agenda may be an unsteady path to change. Janeway (1980) argues that rights are, in fact, only "temporary gifts, granted if the powerful think it desirable but withdrawn at pleasure" (p. 85).

This warning aside, one of the more successful lobby groups for rights protections has been the physically disabled. Discussions of disability typically refer globally to the mentally and physically disabled (Albrecht, 1992; Gadacz, 1994) without regard to potential differences. However, I would argue that there are substantial differences that must be taken into account. First and foremost, the idea of a mental disability usually evokes images of people who are developmentally delayed instead of those with psychiatric diagnoses. Marching under the banner of the mentally disabled is highly likely to net consumers and survivors even further misunderstandings of their public image. In addition, in speaking of both mental and physical disability, Gadacz states that "disability can never be denied" (p. 56) and, indeed, no one can dispute a developmental handicap or the reality of the loss of limbs or eyesight. Yet, almost every aspect of mental illness is contested ground. Some authors even argue that it doesn't exist (Szasz, 1974). In addition, many consumers and survivors may have intermittent episodes of mental or emotional difficulties, but still function fully and healthily most of the time. Others may have had only one "breakdown," never requiring treatment again. In fact, under most circumstances, members of the general public would have no way of identifying consumers and survivors unless they are visibly marked by the side effects of present or past psychiatric medication. Also, although theories about mental illness abound, there is no conclusive agreement on what it is, what causes it or what to do about it. Consequently, as respondents have demonstrated, it's hard to develop a clear advocacy agenda that has the potential of obtaining public and political acceptance. A final and major difference between people with physical disabilities and those who might be said to have a "mental disability" is that, in the latter case, involuntary treatment is sanctioned by law. While the physically disabled may, with justification, complain of the traditionally patriarchal nature of medicine, they retain the right to refuse treatment. But mental patients can have this most basic choice suspended.

Notwithstanding these sorts of blocks to subsuming consumers and survivors under the global term "disabled," many mental health professionals (as discussed in chapter 2), have begun referring to them as "psychiatrically disabled"—an oddly circular designation that seeks to define disability in terms of the medical specialty that diagnoses the problem in the first place. Some consumers and survivors joke that it is, in fact, a more accurate term than most people realize, given their contention that mental patients have been disabled by the psychiatric treatment they receive.

As with physical disabilities, an entire professional field centred on the rehabilitation of the psychiatrically disabled has evolved. Critics of this "rehabilitation industry" (Albrecht, 1992, p. 7) argue that, in imitation of its close cousin, the medical profession, which in Marxian terms is said to "produce" disease, psychiatric rehabilitation specialists produce disability. Just as psychiatric diagnoses create spoiled identities (Goffman, 1963), disability entombs people within an additional layer of a stigmatized social shell constructed of negative and marginalizing attributions. At the same time, it colonizes their identities so that they can be "worked on" by employees of both the medical profession and the more recently minted rehabilitation industry. The role of rehabilitation is to exert a powerful socialization process that first severs people from their personal histories and then redefines them in the language of disability and handicap—a role that is reminiscent of the Foucauldian view of medicine and psychiatry. The skills people learn during the rehabilitation process are those appropriate to being a "good" patient—someone who is easy to manage, dependent and ignorant of his or her rights—an agenda that appears to be the precise opposite of the consumer and survivor vision of a power contract based on self-empowerment and liberating power relations.

When disability is viewed as a product that is manufactured through professional-client relationships, it becomes clear that it is likely to be the professionals who will have almost total control over interactions within the disability power contract (Gadacz, 1994). Physical disability groups have long recognized this imbalance and have demanded changes so that their needs are more fully recognized. While they have similar experiences and similar complaints, their agendas for change seem much more clearly defined than those of consumers and survivors. For example, they demand (not ask, not request, but *demand*) legally sanctioned equality through such vehicles as the Canadian Charter of Rights and Freedoms. They insist on full participation in the planning, monitoring and delivery of services that affect them—and in this case it was *their* idea and not that of well-intentioned professionals. They want integration into the community of their choice and Canadian society as a whole. They also demand to be seen as individuals who must have their personally defined needs and aspirations respected and, finally, they call for systems of accountability, insisting that professionals answer for both their "actions and inactions" (Gadacz, 1994, p. 91). A final point, which is considered to be absolutely central to the physical disability movement, is the "dignity of risk" (p. 80). Physically disabled adults cannot and should not be protected against bad decisions and embarrassing mistakes.

The wider disability movement has some decided appeal for consumers and survivors in that it affords them access to a powerful rights lobby group with a demonstrated track record. However, the reality is that consumers and survivors have felt somewhat on the outside of these groups, unable to make their particular concerns heard. One respondent explains:

> We don't really fit in. Ultimately, society's concept of disability doesn't include people like consumers/survivors. Like, if you have no legs, you have no legs. That doesn't have to be measured. But with mental illness, they get into *how* mentally ill you are and that kind of thing. With physical disabilities, people go, "Aaawh, that's so sad." If you say you have a mental illness, people go, "Oooooh, that's scary." Like the reaction, the stigma of it is different.
>
> The other thing is, just because you have a disability doesn't necessarily make you sensitive to other people's disabilities. I can be just as insensitive to someone with a mobility impairment as they can be to me.
>
> So this disability thing, it just doesn't fit. I write about people with "psychiatric disabilities" only so that I can use the whole human rights argument. I don't consider myself disabled—which is not to say that people who have been labelled mentally ill don't have periods when they need a lot of support.
>
> Another problem is that the only time we interact with other disability groups is around legislative stuff— equity, accommodation, that kind of thing. And, a lot of the things that the rest of the disability movement is fighting for have been decided upon long before we even get to the table. I, myself, wrote about accommodation for psychiatric survivors in colleges and universities. I was aware that it's kind of ludicrous to be writing about accommodations for a group that has an unemployment rate of between 80 and 90%. So, we're talking apples and oranges. I stay in it to kind of keep our foot in the door—just to keep ourselves visible so that we have a voice. But, at the same time, there's an acknowledgment that we're not even close to getting some of the recognition and access that people with disabilities have.

None of the respondents felt that the term disabled could be accurately applied to them. Nevertheless, it carries with it an entrée to some of the things that consumers and survivors value. For example, it assists them in recasting, in civil rights terms, debates over involuntary treatment or community treatment orders. In practical terms, the disability designation also allows access to a somewhat higher rate of social assistance than offered through basic welfare. However, it must also be acknowledged that, while the physically disabled don't have a choice as to whether or not they are going to wrestle with the concept of disability, most consumers and survivors have the option to choose, individually and collectively, to use or, in the end, to abandon this identity marker, judging it to be a path that may possibly offer too few rewards given the uncertain destination to which it leads.

In conclusion

In keeping with the theoretical context of the research, the embryonic ideology of the consumer and survivor movement, at least as it is defined by this study's respondents, centres on power and its uses and abuses in our society. Consumers and psychiatric survivors appear to have fastened on a fundamental set of questions that challenge the foundation of all social relations. Dominance is the basis for most of our present power contracts, from small, local and intensely personal familial relationships to large, worldly social relations that characterize operations in government, politics and the mental health system. Power contracts based on self-empowerment and liberating power relations are currently reasonably rare exceptions to the dominant rule and, given the general invisibility of power that is so much a part of a society founded on principles of hegemonic control, such a fundamental alteration in how we relate to one another remains extremely difficult to institute in the first place and to maintain in the second. Certainly, when consumers and survivors began developing their own organizations, they merely reproduced the damaging power relations they so much feared. But, as Jennifer Chambers so succinctly puts it, "People who've been fucked over are fucked up." When aspirations and visions for the future are painted with the aid of a large philosophical brush, a natural frustration is to search vainly for what, specifically and concretely, consumers and survivors want. Simply but broadly stated, they seem to want a life. However, the necessary and time-consuming precursor to that life is defining their beliefs and values, which will then constitute the rock-hard foundation upon which a more refined advocacy agenda can rest. It is a painful and lengthy process that may take decades to complete.

10

Final thoughts and understandings

This work began with a description of life in a psychiatric hospital where the underlying tenets of the power contract between staff and patients appeared to be straightforward. The patients needed help and we, as professionals, were trained to be helpful. However, each group had a different perception of, first, what was wrong and, second, what to do about it. In the midst of a tense and chaotic ward atmosphere, coupled with community discharge destinations that included poverty and violence, both staff and patients alike seemed to conclude that nothing changes and no one gets better. However, staff-patient relationships were not the only interactions in the hospital that were based on power. Staff, who occupied a position of power in patients' lives, felt themselves to be powerless in the face of administration, often raising many of the same sorts of complaints that the patients had of them. "Our concerns don't matter. We have no say in the decisions that affect our lives." And administration, in its turn, appeared to feel powerless in relation to the Ministry of Health, seeing its representatives as capricious, sometimes punitive and oblivious to the realities they faced.

A review of the history of insanity pointed out that staff and patients of the very same hospital had been having similar experiences for nearly two centuries. Although periods of reform have come and gone, along with a variety of treatment modalities that alternately emphasized nature or nurtured etiological theories, conditions for mental patients have remained pretty much the same. They live outside of society's universe of obligation (Gamson, 1995), exploited and marginalized, feared and fearful, yet consistently asking for the basic human necessities: friends, family, a home and a job.

When society becomes divided into those who are inside the universe of obligation and those who are outside, it creates a duality of thinking that severs and polarizes: powerful and powerless, have and have not, harmed or harming. Gil (1996) views denial of opportunity as a form of initiating social violence, which he defines as a set of actions that constitute the beginning of a three-part spiral of violence. The second part of this spiral is the threat of reactive counter-violence, created when powerless people are unable to meet their own needs, no matter how hard they try. In such an atmosphere, the tendency is for society to both produce and submit to an intricate web of rules and regulations, thereby creating the third part of the spiral, a repressive social response which is itself a form of violence. In the production of his three-part theory, Gil is employing a broadened definition of violence which, in Wartenberg's (1990) terms, relates to all activity, visible and invisible, that produces and maintains dominance. These are the sorts of forces that result in the creation of a power contract based on dominance. Those in power seek control over the less powerful, by force if necessary, employing an "it's for your own good" justification designed to elicit both compliance and gratitude and creating an invisible web of hegemonic control. Both the powerful and the powerless repress their uneasiness and agree that "it's just the way things are."

In the case of mental health and psychiatry, the close confines of the psychiatric ward, the emotional crucible of the family and the mean city streets are examples of initiating social violence that can give way to reactive counter-violence. While incidents of actual violence among mental patients are, in fact, low (Arboleda-Florez, Holley & Crisanti, 1996; Monahan & Arnold, 1996) they are nevertheless accorded a saliency that drives legislation. The power of psychiatric science is backed by a set of laws that sanctions coercion, creating a pathway for institutionalized violent responses in the form of involuntary commitment and forced treatment. The invisible power of hegemony also allows citizens, who would otherwise view themselves as decent people, to ignore widespread and well-documented abuse and violence perpetrated against mental patients at the hands of the community and state (Roeher Institute, 1995) while, paradoxically, producing a government policy that refers to this same group as "survivors" (*Putting People First*, 1993). The interactive spiral of initiating social violence, which denies mental patients the fulfilment of even their most basic human needs (friends, family, a home and a job), followed by a small but salient show of reactive counter-violence which, in its turn, releases the meta-forces of a legislated response (Gil, 1996), creates and reinforces a mental health system which could be said to be structurally violent—in sum, a place where there is the strong potential that nothing will change because no one *can* get better. And so it has been for nearly two centuries.

Power contracts based on concepts of empowerment and liberation appear to be rare in practice but, nonetheless, populate our utopian dreams of the future as evidenced by their regular emphasis in the rhetoric of mental health reform. At the initiation of yet another period of reform, the government of Ontario initially de-emphasized the role of its traditional partners, psychiatrists and other mental health professionals, and, instead, recruited consumers and psychiatric survivors to help with the production of its mental health policies and plans.

Four questions formed the basis of this work: How did ex-mental patients come to redefine themselves as political activists? How did they translate their personal experiences into collective action? What creed or ideology guides their movement's choices? And, finally, how did they define their relationship to government during these "heady" days? In response to the first question, respondents told stories that took the archetypal form of an odyssey. Their experiences transformed them into sadder but wiser people who now know what is *really* going on. Although many respondents eventually received help from a specific psychiatrist or other mental health professional, they interpreted this fact to be merely the exception that proved the rule. In their view, their experiences created a special bond among their fellow travellers, based on a unique form of oppression related to what they think of as the mental health system's attempt to capture their minds and spirits.

In reclaiming and recreating their own identities, respondents relied heavily on the mirror of the Other which, in this case, is composed of mental health professionals. Professionals provided the road map that showed respondents all they should *not* be: fearful of their own emotions, dedicated to the appearance rather than the reality of ethical conduct, contemptuous of the very help they are supposed to be offering, self-interested and, above all, embedded in a web of rigid rules and regulations which leaves them focused on legal rather than moral imperatives. However, upon deeper reflection, respondents concluded that perhaps mental health professionals were more like consumers and survivors than they had at first thought. "Everybody's afraid," says Jennifer Chambers. The phrase, "I'm not in control, there's no money, no support," has become the universal complaint, whether one is a consumer, survivor or a mental health professional.

Respondents were equally candid about their views of their own efforts at collective action and in forming economic development and self-help organizations with funds from the government-sponsored Consumer/Survivor Development Initiative. Respondents used the colourful term "cannibalism" to describe the spate of infighting that sapped their energy and opened fresh wounds. They concluded that it's all about power. Having themselves been terribly hurt by what they view as the misuse of power, they recoiled at its expression within their own ranks. Indeed, their flagship organization, the Ontario Psychiatric Survivors Alliance (OPSA) folded under just this sort of pressure, leaving respondents feeling embarrassed and saddened. While this very public downfall is a living example of what disability groups see as a fundamental human right—the "dignity of risk" (Gadacz, 1994, p. 91)—it nevertheless serves as a reminder that failure, while almost always instructive, is also painful.

On the subject of their new-found partnership status with government, respondents described themselves as both flattered and puzzled, but, above all, suspicious. "It wasn't *our* idea," they said. Nevertheless, they recognized the opportunities inherent in their popularity, but also felt drained by the constant effort to get professionals to listen, the apparent lack of visible change and the disturbing feeling that they had been, in fact, used. They also noticed that the idea of partnership only extended to the point where issues of autonomy and freedom were raised. They concluded that mental health reform, in its present incarnation, could not possibly work because "the power dynamics haven't changed."

In the midst of the pressures from the influx of funds and the government's call for partnership, consumers and survivors failed to distinguish their own advocacy goals as distinct and separate from the many other interests represented in the mental health reform process. While a civil rights agenda may hold some promise, respondents actually concentrated more on the need for what they called emotional and economic supports. To them, emotional support means an emphasis on empathy, guidance and encouragement instead of involuntary commitment, forced medication and electro-convulsive therapy. It also means friends, family and a community. Economic support is defined as a home and a job. Some respondents were optimistic that they would, eventually, be able to achieve their political goals. Others felt that their fragile movement was already drifting apart, having missed an important window of opportunity that was now closed. However, most point out that, although they've been saying the same things for over two centuries, there have always been people who have been "willing to stay in there with their hearts."

So, what's it all about?

The character of qualitative research is to raise questions and stimulate thought more than it is to provide answers. Consequently, I cannot offer even the illusion that I have arrived at a polished set of conclusions. It is also entirely possible that my understandings may differ substantially from those that readers themselves will develop. So, too, will my own thinking evolve, but at this time and in this place the thoughts that follow are my personal take on what it's all about.

A legacy of violence

First, I think it is important to revisit the reality that the story of the mental health system, historically and in its current incarnation, is nothing if not a tale of violence and tragedy. Consumers, survivors, families and professionals see, hear and experience acts of incredible violence no matter what their paradigm or group allegiance may be. The viewpoint that mental illness is exclusively a biological disorder does not protect proponents against witnessing unbearable anguish as people are tormented by the vicious demons of schizophrenia or weighed down by the "black dog" of depression that sentences them to a despair so acute that a vocabulary is yet to be developed that can adequately describe the pain. Family members weep in agony as they stand by, wanting to help but unable to reach through the veil of disease that separates them from the seemingly lost soul that once was their precious child, wife, mother, brother, sister or father. On the other hand, a social causality paradigm means listening as people recount incidents of child rape and torture perpetrated within the confines of what our society anoints as our most precious resource, the family. In this instance, families must choose between retreating into angry and isolating denial or being torn apart by the revelations. Whichever course they take cannot insulate them against their worst fear: that sometime in the near future they may be bowed down by the grief of suicide when their loved one can no longer go on, or, perhaps equally as horrific, forced to watch helplessly as their son or daughter takes to the streets, disoriented, vulnerable and repeatedly the target of physical and sexual assault. If, as patients or ex-patients, people have experienced these things first hand, they may muster a tentative cry for help, but they contend that it is met with more of the same violence as they are forced into institutions where assaults are common and then discharged to housing that may be violent and ghettoized. And it is the clearest reality for people who call themselves survivors that many, many of their peers have not, in fact, survived.

I repeat these realities here because conducting this study has taught me how easy it is for me to allow them to slip away.

Even as I wrote the above passage, I had to remind myself that I was not recounting the violent incidents that have accumulated over a century, a decade or even a year. I was simply talking about the things I dealt with *last month* in my own work as a mental health professional. While Gil's (1996) theories call for a broadened definition of violence so that it can include neglect, abandonment and a denial of opportunity, the violence that is often the common currency of direct service in, or experience of, the mental health system is of the narrowly defined, commonly understood kind—physical, sexual and emotional abuse. As a society, we seem to be collectively amnesic for the violence we both create and endure. In the mental health system, our endorsement of involuntary commitment and forced treatment colours all that we do. Study respondents insist that it is these coercive and violent aspects of psychiatric treatment that *create* survivors, not because all people who identify as survivors have experienced them, although many have, but simply because they exist. While, for good and substantial reason, respondents are unable to see beyond their own experiences of forced treatment and tend only to view psychiatrists who wield these powers as, at best, untrustworthy and, at worst, sadistic, I know from my own point of view that whenever force enters what was supposed to be a helping relationship, everyone is diminished: the community worker or family member who called the police, the psychiatrist who wrote the order, the nurses who tied the patient down in restraints and the patients and staff who witnessed the event. Mary asks, "Is this health care?" This is an absolutely central question. As a mental health professional myself, nothing in my training taught me that force and coercion is helpful, yet I work in a system governed by laws that sanction such measures in the alleged service of the protection of wider society. As consumers and survivors continue to make their presence felt, whether as partners or in the less-friendly role of political activists, the question of coercion requires centre stage in future discussions because it is the foundation upon which the architecture of the present mental health system rests. In Hegelian terms, it is the threat that maintains a power contract based on relationships of dominance and subjugation, relationships which, in contemporary language, are called oppression. The reality is that an "unjust order negatively affects the oppressor as much as, if not more than, the oppressed" (Memmi, as cited in Duerr, 1996). While the entanglement of caring and control is a historical fact of the mental health system, must it also be its future? As we enter an era of community treatment orders, this is a central question.

The power of powerless people

The point of Janeway's work is to point out that powerless people are not, in fact, totally powerless. And, in fact, consumers and survivors have demonstrated themselves to have had a powerful effect on mental health reform planning.

Telling stories is powerful. During the early period of reform, respondents regularly testified at public forums and legislative hearings using well-told, intensely personal and highly emotional stories. Their presentations were all the more powerful if, as consumers and survivors contend, they live in a society that fears the open expression of emotion.

Sheer numbers are powerful. The presence of hundreds of consumers and survivors in the formerly private domains of mental health professionals and Ministry of Health bureaucrats is a powerful signal that change is possible. Their views and their language have begun to seep into formal and informal mental health parlance, and their advocacy efforts have served as a valiant attempt to shift the tone and the tenor of reform plans.

Standing up and yelling is powerful. When they have the opportunity, consumers and survivors continue to publicly berate professionals and bureaucrats who have yet to yell back. While this sort of confrontative style may lose its shock value over time, so far it seems to be serving its purpose—consumers and survivors are having their say, *fortissimo*.

However, these sorts of victories, important though they may be, are largely symbolic, and respondents have declined to celebrate them, viewing planning for change, as compared with actually making change, as two different things. In addition, they say that they have been used, co-opted by the government's own cost-cutting agenda while the majority of their number remain mired in poverty and degradation. Historical evidence indicates that they are right. While the mental health system has repeatedly attempted its own reform, positive outcomes have been sporadic and short-lived, rapidly deteriorating into the same humiliation and violence they were supposed to alleviate. The government's early policy of "partnership" meant that consumers and survivors spent endless hours involved in planning exercises focused on system management and administrative issues. Yet they profess themselves to be much more interested in practicalities such as housing, employment and education, fundamental components of the social fabric that have suffered substantial erosion under the current Conservative government. Consumers and survivors also seem concerned with the quality and nature of what, for them, is the system's most salient power contract, the professional-patient relationship. It is here, in this intimate and private space, where help in the desired form of empowerment and liberation does, or does not, occur. In the vernacular, it's where the rubber hits the road, and so far there has been little discussion about actual change in this albeit micro but highly critical power contract. Finally, consumers and survivors exhibit an urgency that is not shared by professionals and bureaucrats. While one respondent acknowledges that reform is likely to be a long, long process, spanning much more than just 5 or 10 years, others say, "Unless you *do* something [soon] . . . I'll be dead" (Church, 1996, p. 33).

The literature predicts that movements such as the one that consumers and survivors are attempting to create are likely to experience internal strife. They are also highly vulnerable to a variety of unhappy fates, with co-option being only one possibility. But even though most respondents *know* they are going through the rather predictable ups and downs most movements experience, awareness has little protective power. They still suffer and they do, indeed, struggle—in the fullest Foucauldian sense of the word. As Hugh Tapping says, "Just because you have all the insight in the world doesn't mean it's necessarily going to help." Knowledge must be coupled with skills, and followed by effective action. It is important to recall that advocacy is, by definition, the art of persuading powerful others to change. Self-help, conversely, focuses primarily on interpersonal growth and skills development, with social change emerging as an important but only secondary goal. Strong self-help groups provide a protective shelter for the creation of self-esteem, confidence and pride. They also spawn committed advocates who can do battle effectively in the larger and more dangerous political arena, but only because they are imbued with the sure and certain knowledge that they have the support of their peers and the comfort of a welcoming home base to which they can return. Chamberlin (1978, 1990) is adamant that the establishment of a powerful self-help network is essential to consumers' and survivors' well-being, both individually and collectively. I agree. Certainly, one of the great regrets expressed by this study's respondents is that consumers and survivors don't "stick together." Indeed, effective advocacy depends on solidarity. But solidarity can only arise out of repeated opportunities to spend time in the company of one's peers, and in circumstances that assure freedom from outside influence. The government's creation of the Consumer/Survivor Development Initiative (CSDI) may be the harbinger of a thriving self-help network. However, as respondents point out, government funds come with "strings attached." The inability of consumers and survivors to work productively with this reality was one of the factors that led to the demise of their provincial organization, the Ontario Psychiatric Survivors Alliance (OPSA). In her review of the events that led up to the defunding of OPSA, Shimrat (1997) attempts to put a brave face on disaster, but no inventory of good intentions and "almost" accomplishments can make up for this critical loss. Without the protection and leadership of a central rallying point, the consumer and survivor advocacy agenda may not make much of a lasting impression in the halls of power.

However, with loss comes opportunity. The moment has come for reorientation to the movement's original roots. In order for self-help to succeed unequivocally, there must be a clear, emphatic and independent commitment to its ethos—one that arises solely from within the ranks of consumers and survivors themselves. The results of this work suggest that the government's clarion call to partnership diverted activists away from the most important task, building a solid foundation for their movement. Now may be the time to return to this basic task.

The powerlessness of powerful people

The concept of power contract is designed to point out the power of powerless people. It does not, however, account for the powerlessness of powerful people—the thousands of mental health professionals who appear to be the primary target of respondents' ire. While on occasion I have been similarly critical of my own and others' professional roles in the mental health system, I nonetheless found myself moved to sympathy for my beleaguered colleagues.

There is unquestionable substance to the criticism respondents level at workers in the mental health system. However, I noted that consumers and survivors recognized their own sense of fear and powerlessness reflected in the demeanour of the mental health professionals from whom they had received service in the past or with whom, in the present, they share membership on boards, committees and planning groups. Mental health professionals, respondents say, are just as afraid as they are. Certainly, this view is consistent with my own experience where I observed that power relationships based on dominance are the norm in the rigidly hierarchical, top-down organizational structures in which most professionals work. Workers who themselves feel frightened, disregarded and disempowered are predictably vulnerable to reproducing these same conditions among their own patients and clients. In addition, professionals are constrained by the formal and informal rules and regulations that are the price of membership in the inner circle of power. They eschew bad manners and, instead, swallow their anger (Church, 1996). While they have tried to insist that consumers and survivors might benefit from being "nice" (Melville Whyte, 1996, p. 22), consumers and survivors, in their turn, aren't buying it. Anger, they say, is a natural and healthy response to oppression, and its expression is liberating. This is valuable advice for mental health professionals who are themselves suffering their own form of oppression.

As long as professionals work in a system that supports dominance, their ability to be helpful in the way that consumers and survivors are demanding is limited. Powerless people simply cannot empower and liberate. One of the clearest findings of the present research is that respondents do not agree with Thomas Szasz (1974) when he asserts that mental illness is a myth. Instead, they describe deep suffering and a desperate longing for help. Mental health professionals want to help. However, professionals who themselves lack the emotional support of empathy, guidance and encouragement are predictably unable to offer these same comforts to their patients and clients. In short, while the majority of mental health professionals remain frightened and disempowered, it is possible that nothing *will* change because no one *can* get better—surely the most costly and ineffective strategy of all.

Things change and people get better

Perhaps the most important revelation of this research lies in the briefly mentioned and easily missed fact that many respondents reported that they actually found help within the confines of the formal mental health system, and it was provided by a mental health professional. However, respondents moved swiftly over this revelation, pursuing, in preference, impassioned discussions of where and how the system failed. Given their political role, it is understandable that their focus is on what's wrong, rather than on what's right. The helpers of whom respondents speak so favourably exit quickly from the narrative stage, leaving the impression that receiving help from a mental health professional is nothing but a lucky accident. And perhaps, within the broader terrain of the mental health system, this view is accurate. However, I can't help but want to know more. What can be learned from these instances? Within the confines of the present work, it can only be documented that they occur. Regrettably, this is only a faint beacon, but its importance should not be minimized. Prevailing wisdom, often propounded both at a professional and at a lay level, identifies a diagnosis of mental illness as a life-long burden, sentencing sufferers to the bleakest of futures characterized only by decline. The respondents in this study each received such a sentence, yet they stand as living proof that things *do* change and people *can* get better. From the perspective of this work, exactly by what process this miracle occurs remains a mystery.

A political identity in search of a future

The final understanding that I take from my research experience concerns both the opportunities and the limitations of "psychiatric survivor" as a political identity. All study respondents rejected the professionally generated term consumer, preferring instead the more militant identity of survivor. Indeed, the term psychiatric survivor figured prominently in Ontario mental health policy, for reasons that are perhaps the government's own, but nonetheless its presence formally acknowledged a group of people who believe that psychiatric treatment, as it is currently constituted, is the punishing instrument through which survivors are created. The utility of the survivor identity is as a political tool. It valorizes the suffering that people have endured and connects it to a specific cause. It politicizes individual experience by illuminating the oppressive social structures that create stigma, marginalization, violence and poverty—experiences which, indeed, can only be survived. However, to be a survivor, even a publicly acknowledged one, is to embrace an identity without an obvious future, despite its strong past. The word means, in its standard definition, to have made it through, to have outlasted the threat. But then what? There is no vision that extends beyond this horizon.

Having escaped once is erroneously thought to provide added confidence, in that survivors now know that they could make it through again, should they once more be tested. However, as study respondents have pointed out, ignorance provides its own protection. In fact, "knowing" can become a formidable enemy because its legacy is fear. One of the greatest concerns for respondents is the fear of retaliation. Could they survive a second time? I didn't sense that respondents believed that they could. As a result, the survivor identity may offer only the appearance of power and, like whistling in the dark, protect only so long as the enemy believes in its strength.

Finally, one respondent states, "I want to do more than just survive." While no one can deny the initial experience of liberation that the adoption of the survivor identity seems to provide, there is nevertheless the possibility that, without careful reflection and management, it may become claustrophobic over time, especially in its less-manoeuvrable collective expression. The current and pressing challenge for the consumer and psychiatric survivor movement is to develop a shared ideology that clearly describes their advocacy agenda. While it is true that their movement is in its infancy and may struggle with this task for many years to come, a logical but perhaps unrecognized first step along the developmental voyage may well be a strategy for exiting from the conceptual confines of their own survivor identity. "It's hard for people to even imagine something different," says Jennifer Chambers, and in this she may be correct. The future for consumers and survivors seems to rest in a place where presently it cannot be imagined, and their difficult task is to reach beyond "just surviving" towards a clarity of vision and purpose that will guide and sustain their movement. To fail to do so will only leave them rudderless and vulnerable, the regressive and all-too-familiar state from which many movement members have only just emerged.

In conclusion

The field of mental health has effectively resisted reform for over two centuries, creating, over and over again, conditions under which, it is often said, nothing changes and no one gets better. The reality is that the mental health system is both the creation and the creator of the same forces that govern the society in which it is embedded. Presently, society itself is changing. Traditional power relationships are re-forming themselves in response to an explosion in both the amount and availability of knowledge. As the powerful lose their exclusive grip on the production and distribution of knowledge, an opening is created for substantial, worldwide change. The long-term path to altering our inherently violent society is the support and nurturance of non-violent liberation movements such as the one consumers and survivors are struggling to create. The goal of this new type of social movement is the emancipation of both the powerful and the powerless through the production and maintenance of new relationships based on empowerment and liberation. Study respondents state that they have found a healthy outlet for their anger. In doing so, they have begun a journey that can only benefit us all.

Postscript

(May 2000)

As an observer of, and participant in, the production of the past decade's contribution to the lineage of mental health history, I have occupied a front-row seat for the political, bureaucratic and professional drama in which the consumer and survivor movement has played its role. At the time of writing, mental health reform planning seems to be reaching some sort of conclusion, fully 12 years after the publication of the Graham Report. During this time, Ontario has experienced the full spectrum of political leadership available to the electorate. The reform process began during the reign of a Liberal government, picked up speed while the New Democrats were in power and stands on the threshold of implementation at a time when a Conservative government has been given its second mandate. The rapid swings in political sentiment—from middle, to left and then to right—represent a recession-weary public's search for a simple answer to their woes. Indeed, it appears that the Conservatives have been most successful in this task, riding to power in 1995 on a platform composed of the "common-sense revolution" and repeating this feat in 1999 with its similarly toned Blueprint. The common-sense revolution laid the blame for the province's miseries at the feet of a bloated, self-interested public service that had aided and abetted former governments in a headlong rush into fiscal debt. It also identified welfare as an excessive and often larcenous drain on the public purse. And the electorate agreed, giving the Conservatives two majority governments in succession.

In its first term, the Conservative government instituted billions of across-the-board cuts to public spending, cutting back welfare payments by 21.6%, while, at the same time, reducing personal income tax by 15%. Health care, however, had been considered sacrosanct. The Conservatives promised that the $17.4 billion[1] in health spending inherited from the previous government would remain intact. The lay public initially interpreted this promise as a commitment to the status quo. This was not the case. Within this funding envelope, wide-ranging changes were planned. A government-appointed Health Services Restructuring Commission swept across the province, directing substantial hospital closures and recommending the divestment of 9 out of the 10 provincial psychiatric hospitals. All programs previously provided by these institutions were to be transferred to public hospitals and then, in most cases, downsized.

Another round of mental health planning resulted in one more report, called *2000 and Beyond* (Newman, 1998). Its stated goal was to re-evaluate *Putting People First* "to identify areas where improvements are needed" (p. 30). Extensive consultation confirmed the need for adding to community services before the psychiatric hospitals are downsized—but there was one addition that had never been part of previous plans. Extensive and persistent family lobbying has convinced the government to review the Mental Health Act to "ensure the effectiveness of the legislation" (p. 6). This review is in direct response to family and general public belief that the current Act focuses too heavily on individual liberties and should be revised to give psychiatrists increased powers to treat patients on an involuntary basis and to write community treatment orders. Such measures represent a significant defeat for consumers and survivors.

To date, the Consumer/Survivor Development Initiative's budget has remained intact and, while it could be argued that it has but a slim toehold in the overall mental health funding arena, an early evaluation of the program demonstrated that its many self-help and economic development projects have contributed to a reduction in the length and frequency of stays in hospital for their members, and, further, physician's visits and crisis contacts were down (Trainor et al., as cited in Wilson,

---

1 In the run-up to the election of June 3, 1999, this spending level was increased to $20.7 billion for the fiscal year 1999/2000.

1996). However, there have been some disasters among the successes, and they provide ample fodder for closing down the entire project—should the government so wish. Currently, it is my impression that the continued existence of the initiative depends more on the maintenance of a low, non-offensive profile than it does on the solidification of a strong power base.

Individually, consumers and survivors have been hard hit by cuts to welfare and the allowances paid to single mothers. In addition, changes in rent control legislation and a proposed shift to local municipalities of the responsibility for subsidized housing may mean that further hardships are forthcoming.[2] While the vacillating political climate has produced chaos in the formal mental health service sector, frightening professionals and bureaucrats even more than was the case when reform was originally proposed, paradoxically, it has also created a peaceful moment for consumers and survivors. The intense pressure of "partnership" has abated. The faint but rallying scent of betrayal is once again in the air, and Pat Capponi, a prominent survivor leader, seems to have regained her angry edge. She writes:

> I assumed that all we needed to do was expose conditions and government would be forced to act. I kept that belief, and it kept me, for over 17 years, years of meetings with ministers of health, bureaucrats by the handful, and mental health professionals. It was often brutal, frustrating, every psychiatric survivor's death a failure I wore personally. I hadn't done enough to let people know. But I believed, you see, and my community believed in me. (Capponi, 1996, p. 17)

While it remains true that consumers and survivors continue to be recruited for Boards of Directors and the occasional committee meeting, their participation in most aspects of the mental health system is no longer actively sanctioned by government. More subtly, the involvement they retain has become much less of a disturbing novelty. Habituation carries with it its own threat. Repetition tends to de-fang once sharply con-

---

2 Prior to the June 1999 election, the Conservative government announced $45 million for housing specifically for the homeless and the mentally ill.

frontative critiques, and a ubiquitous presence can become a recipe for a new form of invisibility, one born of familiarity.

The last word belongs to the consumers and survivors who have populated these pages. Throughout this work, they have professed themselves to be optimistic, pessimistic, cynical, hopeful, weary, afraid, lonely, embattled, empowered, disgusted and puzzled, but I note that they never used terms like bored or defeated. In conclusion, each offers their own view of what the future holds.

Susan Marshall:

> I think sometime soon, I'm going to have to move on—to what, I'm not sure, but I think I'll always be involved in some way.

Jennifer Reid:

> I think we're going to end up divided. The grass-roots activists are going to clash with the middle-class activists and we're going to have so much infighting that the government is going to be able to implement any type of law it wants, and by the time we quit fighting about it—it will be all over with.

Marilyn Nearing:

> I'm probably going to be involved until I die because why would I give up something that gives me such joy? I am hopeful that there will be pockets of success that we can build on. People have obtained a wellness through this . . . and we have a lot of dynamic leaders out there. And you know, it's really strange, but I think there might be a chance after the economy being so bad and everyone's job being threatened, there might be an opportunity for the general public to identify with us because so many of them are in a position of vulnerability.

(Special note: Marilyn did, indeed, remain involved until she died. Sadly, in May 1999, she passed away from cancer.)

Paul Reeve:

> If they cut the funding to our CSDI programs, people will have to search out other types of jobs just to survive and that puts a lid on things. I think there could be a future,

but I recognize the need for financial support to ensure that future.

Mary:

> There will always be some die-hards who will remain committed. They may need to take time out now and again, but there will always be people pushing for change.

Marg Oswin:

> The window of opportunity that we had—the glory days—the days of the Graham Report in the late '8os when we thought anything was possible—that window has closed. I think we're entering a period of withdrawal from the field. We're resting, learning from our mistakes and preserving our hope for the future. It's still there. Every time we get together in a group, I feel a bond, a unity, an enthusiasm that's always there. That's not gone anywhere. We're just hibernating right now, but we're still alive. I think another opportunity will come and we'll be better able to deal with it. It would be nice if it happened in my lifetime. I don't know if it will . . . but as long as people are oppressed, they'll rise up and fight it.

Donna:

> I think we're drifting apart. Consumers and consumer groups are isolated from one another. The funding has never been adequate. There are a lot of movements that grow without funding, but I don't think this is going to be one of them. And we all have different agendas for change. I would like to say that I see this as a challenge but I don't. I see it as the thing that will cause this particular movement to fizzle out. We had our chance and we missed it.

A respondent who preferred anonymity:

> You can't erase people. You can put them down in one place, but they pop up somewhere else. If you go look at the archives at Queen Street, you'll see that survivors at the turn of the century were writing letters and asking the same questions. "Hey, I worked in the laundry for 15 years, how come I never got paid?" Letters from the *turn of the century* saying the same thing that we're saying now. You can't silence people because it always comes up in some

other, more subversive way. I tend to look at things in a really broad timeline. Like, I'm not really thinking about the next 5 or 10 years. I don't have a vision of the end . . . what it's going to look like. I also tend not to worry about the unity of the movement because I don't necessarily feel that unity is a good thing. I think people's individual voices get drowned out. So, I'm the kind of person who shrugs and waits to see what will happen. I do my best in my corner of the world, and if I have an opportunity to effect some change, I do it.

Sue Goodwin:

Well, our future is going to be different than the past. I don't know if it's going to be better. I hear voices out there in places that I wouldn't expect to hear them and what we have to say isn't such a cry in the wilderness as it used to be. We're out there. We're trading information on things that are happening in Toronto, the States and even the Yukon. And we're all saying the same thing, just in different words. The little dribble of funding we got from the government helped our movement to form, but it's not going to keep us surviving. We have to find our own funding. We're not going away.

Walter Osoka:

I need to get a job. I'm on unemployment right now. But I'd like to take part as a board member or a volunteer, whatever, as long as I can.

Dave Stewart:

Psychiatry is not an easy thing to take power from and as liberal as certain professionals sound, they have a lot to protect and they will protect it. But I don't think you can quite get us to go away. Look at the women's movement and all the trouble they've had. You can't stop these things once they've established some history; you can't stop them completely. And we have our own bit of history now.

Hugh Tapping:

We can't be defeated as long as the system is as nasty as it is. It will keep manufacturing new versions of survivors.

John:

> I think we've come a long way. Our organizations have proved a lot. Ten or 15 years ago, the movement, if there was a movement, didn't have any real resources. I think things will get better unless the Ministry relaxes things and ignores its own guidelines for consumer participation on Boards and committees.

Patrick Brown:

> I don't want to do this for the rest of my life. Chances are that in the next five or six years, I'll be moving on. My ultimate goal is to go overseas and do community development work.

M.:

> It would be interesting if I could just fly off somewhere and come back in 10 years and see what's happening. It's fragmented right now. There are all these rivalries and jealousies. It's all tied up with power and money.

Marnie Shepherd:

> All movements go through these things. We have got to spend time thinking about what's going right with our organizations so that we don't become caught up in everything that's going wrong. I can go visit our CSDI groups and they have things going horrifically wrong with them at the board and staff levels, but I sit down to coffee with a member coming in the door—which is why the group exists in the first place—and he just thinks everything is hunky-dory. It's not as bad as we think it is. There might be organizational trouble, but the people who want to use the organization—the members—what they need is still there.

Adele Rosenbloom:

> I really hope that survivors can come together and create a movement that *will* enable real change to take place. I hope we can learn to support each other and give each other the kind of respect we need so that we can work together. I see it happening in small ways.

Jennifer Chambers:

> My hope is that the movement will develop an independent
> vision of what we want to have happen so that mental
> health reform doesn't end up being an endless series of
> tiny variations of what we have now . . . so that there will
> be some actual, real, life-changing alternatives developed
> so that we can see that it doesn't have to be the way it is
> now. People need to start thinking from the bottom up . . .
> which will probably never happen within the Ministry of
> Health. People have to be willing to give up the false pro-
> tection of psychiatry if they want to move forward.

Jane Pritchard:

> I'm very good at old sayings and one of them is "right is
> might." We're not going to go away quietly. In fact, we are
> not going to go away *at all*. This is our fight! This isn't
> about their jobs! This is about dignity and respect and the
> right to a life. So, you know me, boy, don't fuck with me
> when I believe I am right. I'm not going away and there are
> a lot more just like me.

Appendix I
Research methodology

Sample selection

Twenty people were approached and asked to participate in the research. As is typical of qualitative research, the
size of the sample is of less concern than its depth, which is
defined as the importance of working longer and more
intensely with a few people rather than interviewing many in a
brief and superficial manner. The sample is not intended to
represent the rest of the world, but to provide an opportunity
to understand specifically the life-worlds of only this study's
respondents (McCracken, 1990).

A concern related to sampling is that of access—how
the researcher contacts her respondents and gains their co-
operation. In the case of this work, access was less problematic
than it might have been because I knew of some of the respondents through my work. Nevertheless, I was aware that many
consumers and psychiatric survivors feel that they have been
"studied to death" in clinical contexts and resent yet another
researcher taking up their time. Thus, I employed the snowball
method of recruiting, with many respondents offering one or
two additional names of people they thought might be interested in participating. An advantage of this technique was that
I was able to introduce myself to many informants by stating
that a previous interviewee had suggested that I call. I found
that this form of introduction, aside from simply being a polite
way of entering the consumer and survivor network, lent both
me and my work credibility. It is important to note that I did
not employ any specific method that dictated which recommendations I pursued and which I did not. In fact, most of the

names I received led me to willing participants, with only one individual proving herself to be completely unreachable.

I employed no other selection criteria than that the respondents in question identified as consumers or survivors and that they were currently active in what is being termed the "movement." I did, however, ask that people be willing to speak to "big-picture" issues as well as individual experiences so that I would be able to discuss a spectrum of topics and concerns. In other words, I wanted our discussions to range from the personal to the political.

My sampling technique serendipitously delivered a reasonable selection of men and women consumers and survivors (6 men and 13 women), but I had to actively recruit people from areas of the province other than Toronto in service of providing a rural or small-town perspective versus a large urban one. Seven of the interviewees were from outside the city.

Eventually, 20 respondents were interviewed. However, one withdrew permission to use her interview due to involvement in child custody proceedings where it was felt that even an anonymous presentation of her experiences would jeopardize her case.

A global view of the respondents

Basic statistics

Age	Married or common law	Divorced or sepa- rated	Single	Em- ployed	Unem- ployed	Inpa- tient	Out- patient only
32-59	5	5	9	13[a]	6	16	3

a As a brief note, the average level of employment for people with histories of mental illness is between 10 and 15% (Anthony, 1994) while this sample reaches the 68% level.

Out of the 19 respondents, 9 were single, 5 were married or living common law, 1 was separated and 4 were divorced. They ranged in age from 32 to 59. Seven were employed through CSDI projects, 4 in other consumer and survivor initiatives with different sources of funding, 2 were working as direct service providers in the mental health system, 4 were on some form of social assistance and 2 did not work but had private means of support. Three of the respondents had been treated only on an outpatient basis and had not experienced hospitalization.

It was also important to understand the extent of respondents' involvement with the mental health system. The 16 respondents with inpatient histories had spent a total of 256.25 months in institutions, or approximately 21 years. Lengths of admission ranged from 2 weeks to 5 years, with 16 months as the average length of stay and 10 1/2 months as the mean. Two respondents had spent less than a month in hospital, 5 had spent from 1 to 6 months, 1 from 6 months to a year, 5 from 1 to 2 years, 2 from 2 to 3 years and one had spent a total of 5 years in hospital.

Length of inpatient experience (16 respondents)

Total	Range	Average	Mean
12 years	2 weeks to 5 years	16 months	10 1/2 months

In addition, I asked respondents about their psychiatric diagnoses. Three respondents said that they had had so many diagnoses that they didn't know what the final verdict was, 1 didn't complete that portion of the questionnaire, 7 listed their multiple diagnoses, which included borderline personality disorder, depression and schizophrenia, 2 were diagnosed with manic-depression, 4 with depression alone, 1 with schizophrenia and 1 with a form of dissociative disorder.

Psychiatric diagnoses

Multiple diagnoses	Manic-depression	Depression	Schizophrenia	Dissociative disorder	Didn't know or didn't say
7	2	4	1	1	4

Data collection techniques and sources

The primary source of data was 19 in-depth interviews lasting from 1 to 2 hours and conducted over a 2-year period. I taped all interviews and then transcribed them, producing written texts for analysis. The interview setting was in the location of the respondent's choice: at my office, at their office or home, at a coffee shop or bar. In the case of out-of-town interviewees, I spoke with respondents over the telephone, using a special recording device. The main concern was that people felt at ease and not under any time pressure. To that end, some respondents asked to see the questions in advance so that they might think over their answers while others made no such request. In addition, when conducting face-to-face interviews, I always had a copy of the interview questions available for respondents to refer to as the interview progressed. Although this courtesy is a relatively small gesture, this group of people has made it clear that they distrust pieces of paper in the hands of mental health professionals because they have so often been assured that documents such as commitment forms, court assessments, child custody papers and so on were innocuous, only to find out that, in fact, they had life-shattering consequences.

I employed a semi-structured interview guide which listed 12 to 13 questions, some of which were revised or added in light of the data produced as the study progressed. For example, I used the first set of questions for 3 interviews, revised them slightly for 6 more interviews and then revised them once again for the final 10 interviews. Some of the revisions were simply a refinement so that it was abundantly clear what I was asking. As the results section of my work demonstrates, other questions had to be dropped because respondents considered them irrelevant to their experience. And finally, a few questions were added because respondents raised a number of important topics that I had not anticipated.

In addition to 19 interviews, I collected consumer and survivor writings that were published in a variety of forms (newsletters, books, videos, papers, letters to the editor and so on). I also "surfed the Net" for survivor-designed Web pages which, as Toffler (1990) predicted, are becoming ever more prevalent. These further sources of information were adjunctive to the main body of data and were useful for providing background and depth to the respondents' comments.

I also kept a journal throughout the research process where I recorded my thoughts regarding the literature I was reviewing as context for the research, the theoretical perspectives which I felt were applicable, as well as my reactions to the ideas brought out by the various interviews. The journal is a record of my efforts to make sense of what I was reading and hearing and, as such, forms an extremely rough, unorganized and unpolished version of the study as a whole.

Data analysis

Given the nature of my respondents, I felt it extremely important to the trust-building process that I return transcribed interviews to them for verification because consumers and survivors often describe incidents where they feel that their words and experiences have been appropriated for professional gain. Once respondents were satisfied that the transcribed interviews accurately reflected their views in every detail, and they had offered me signed permission to use their words, I felt that I "owned" the data. As a result, the data analysis techniques and the interpretations that result are my productions and, thus, my responsibility.

However, almost all respondents asked that any quotations I chose from their transcript be altered to reflect good grammar, full sentences and a logical flow of ideas. Given that the interviews had been transcribed verbatim, capturing every word that was said, respondents, many of whom are seasoned public speakers or published writers, were shocked at how verbal exchanges "sounded" when they were read. They found the common currency of energetic conversation—examples of which are run-on sentences, inverted logic, incorrect verb tenses, missing words (where gestures had stood in), repetitions, ubiquitous statements of "you know" and verbal ticks like "uhmmmm"—not at all in keeping with the standard of communication to which they aspired. Thus, in deference to their clear, specific and multiple requests, I have altered the quotations that I use for conciseness, flow, readability and grammar—but not for content or meaning.

The first step in the analysis phase of the research was to read and reread the data to ensure complete familiarity. In the case of this work, I transcribed the interviews myself, which gave me a second opportunity to re-experience each one, a helpful, although time-consuming, option that allowed for an increased understanding of the data. In fact, hearing, but not seeing each interview allowed me to concentrate on tone, and I was surprised at the power of the emotion in most respondents' voices, which had been more muted in the actual interview when I was distracted by such sight cues as body language and facial expression.

I chose not to employ a computer program that codes the textual data line by line. Instead, I relied on a manual method, the first step of which was to sort the text by answers to the semi-structured interview questions, devising memos which were, in essence, topic inventories from which categories or themes began to emerge. As familiarity with the data progressed, I began to settle on five categories, each of which constitutes a chapter in the results section of the present work. I then reread the entire data set using only these categories or themes as coding tools. I marked each line or set of lines with a marker pen, the colour of which corresponded to one of the five categories. I found it extremely helpful to be able to visually locate my themes in each interview. The colours pointed out whether or not the themes remained consistent over all 19 interviews. I was also able to see if one or more interviews concentrated on a few themes to the exclusion of others, or if blocks of text within an interview could not be fitted into a theme. These kinds of visual cues allowed me to refine my category titles until all five began to capture most of the data in the majority of the interviews. Closure of this part of the data analysis was achieved when the categories seemed saturated, meaning that the respondents were saying the same or similar things over and over again.

Also, during this process I checked each category for internal homogeneity, looking for contradictions or negative instances—examples of when the theme did not hold true. When contradictions were found, the theme had to be refined even further, often involving a more accurate category title so that it more closely fit the data set. I also reread my other sources of data in the service of external heterogeneity—independent knowledge of the consistency of my categories as compared with other examples of consumer and survivor writings, my own journal and so on. At this point, data analysis began to near completion. The five categories were remaining stable, and I felt I had the basis for describing the life-worlds of my respondents.

References

Agger, B. (1991). Critical theory, poststructuralism, postmodernism: Their sociological relevance. *Annual Review of Sociology, 17,* 105-131.

Akernecht, E. (1968). *A short history of psychiatry.* New York: Hafner Publishing.

Albrecht, G. (1992). *The disability business: Rehabilitation in America.* Newbury Park, CA: Sage Publications.

Anthony, W., Cohen, M., & Farkas, M. (1990). *Psychiatric rehabilitation.* Boston, MA: Centre for Psychiatric Rehabilitation.

Arboleda-Florez, J., Holley, H., & Crisanti, A. (1996). *Mental illness and violence: Proof or stereotype.* (Available from Health Promotions and Programs Branch, Health Canada, Ottawa, ON)

Archer, M. (1990). Human agency and social structure: A critique of Giddens. In J. Clarke, C. Modgil & S. Modgil (Eds.), *Anthony Giddens: Consensus and controversy.* New York: Farmer Press.

Armstrong, P., & Armstrong, H. (1996). *Wasting away: The undermining of Canadian health care.* Toronto, ON: Oxford University Press.

Aronowitz, S. (1992). *The politics of identity: Class, culture, social movements.* New York: Routledge.

Ayd, F., & Blackwell, B. (Eds.). (1970). *Discoveries in biological psychiatry.* Toronto, ON: J.B. Lippincott.

Baird, G. (undated). *999 Queen: A collective failure of imagination.* Article obtained through the Griffin and Greenland Archives. Toronto, ON: The Centre for Addiction and Mental Health.

Bayin, A. (1993, September). Falsely accused. *Homemakers,* pp. 45-52.

Beauvoir, S. de. (1949). *The second sex.* New York: Vintage Books.

Beck, J., & van der Kolk, B. (1987). Reports of childhood incest and current behavior of chronically hospitalized psychotic women. *American Journal of Psychiatry, 144*(1), 1474-1476.

Beers, C. (1908). *A mind that found itself*. New York: Longmans, Green.

Beiser, M. (1990). An update on the epidemiology of schizophrenia. *Canadian Journal of Psychiatry, 35*, 657-688.

Berger, P. (1977). *Facing up to modernity: Excursions in society, politics and religion*. New York: Basic Books.

Blom, D., & Sussman, J. (1989). *Pioneers of mental health and social change, 1930-1989*. London, ON: Third Eye.

Boudreau, F. (1990). *Stakeholders or partners? The roots and challenges of a new politically powerful concept in mental health*. Victoria, BC: Paper presented at the 25th annual meeting of the Canadian Sociological and Anthropological Association.

Boudreau, F., & Lambert, P. (1993a). Compulsory community treatment? I. Ontario stakeholders' response to "helping those who won't help themselves." *Canadian Journal of Community Mental Health, 12*(1), 57-78.

Boudreau, F., & Lambert, P. (1993b). Compulsory community treatment? II. The collision of views and complexities involved: Is it "the best possible alternative"? *Canadian Journal of Community Mental Health, 12*(1), 79-96.

Boydell, K. (1996). *Mothering adult children with schizophrenia: The hidden realities of caring*. Unpublished doctoral dissertation, York University, Toronto, ON.

Breggin, P. (1991). *Toxic psychiatry*. New York: St. Martin's Press.

Browne, G., & Finkelhor, D. (1986). Impact of child sexual abuse: A review of the research. *Psychological Bulletin, 99*(1), 66-77.

Bruner, J. (1995). Meaning and self in cultural perspective. In D. Bakhurst & C. Sypnowich (Eds.), *The social self*. Thousands Oaks, CA: Sage Publications.

Bryer, J., Nelson, B., Miller, J.B., & Krol, P. (1987). Childhood sexual and physical abuse as factors in adult psychiatric illness. *American Journal of Psychiatry, 144*(1), 1426-1430.

Burstow, B. (1992). *Radical feminist therapy: Working in the context of violence*. Newbury Park, CA: Sage Publications.

Canniff, W. (1894). *The medical profession in Upper Canada*. Toronto, ON: William Briggs.

Capponi, D. (1992). *Keynote address*. Presented at the Consumer/Survivor Development Initiative Conference, Toronto, ON.

Capponi, P. (1992a). *Upstairs at the crazy house*. Toronto, ON: Viking Books.

Capponi, P. (Panel member). (1992b). *Meeting the needs*. Symposium conducted at the Conference sponsored by Sistering, Toronto, ON.

Capponi, P. (1996, February 22-28). A lesson for Mike Harris. *NOW Magazine, 15*(25), 17.

Carling, P. (1995). *Return to community: Building support systems for people with psychiatric disabilities*. New York: The Guilford Press.

Carrol, H. (1964). *Mental hygiene: The dynamics of adjustment*. Englewood Cliffs, NJ: Prentice Hall.

Cassin, C. (1993). A psychiatric survivor's challenge. In G. Duplessis, M. McCrea, C. Viscoff & S. Doupe (Eds.), *What works! Innovation in community mental health and addiction treatment programs* (pp. 373-380). Toronto, ON: Canadian Scholars Press.

Cedar Glen home fallout: Government being sued. (1990, July 17). *The Packet and Times*. (Available from the municipal library, Orillia, ON)

Certeau, M. de. (1984). *The practice of everyday life*. Berkeley, CA: The University of California Press.

Chamberlin, J. (1978). *On our own: Patient-controlled alternatives to the mental health system*. New York: Hawthorn Books.

Chamberlin, J. (1990). The ex-patients' movement: Where we've been and where we're going. *The Journal of Mind and Behaviour, 11*(3), 323-336.

Chesler, P. (1972). *Women and madness*. New York: Avon Books.

Chu, J., & Dill, D. (1990). Dissociative symptoms in relation to childhood physical and sexual abuse. *American Journal of Psychiatry, 147*(7), 887-892.

Church, K. (1992). *Moving over*. Toronto, ON: Psychiatric Survivor Leadership Facilitation Program.

Church, K. (1993). *Breaking down/breaking through: Multi-voiced narratives on psychiatric survivor participation in Ontario's community mental health system*. Unpublished doctoral dissertation, University of Toronto, Toronto, ON.

Church, K. (1996). Beyond "bad manners": The power relations of "consumer participation" in Ontario's community mental health system. *Canadian Journal of Community Mental Health, 15*(2), 27-44.

Church, K., with Capponi, Pat. 1991. *Re/membering ourselves: A resource book on psychiatric survivor leadership facilitation.* (Available from the Gerstein Centre, Toronto, ON)

Cohen, S. (1985). *Visions of social control: Crime, punishment and classification.* Cambridge, MA: Polity Press.

Collins, A. (1988). *In the sleep room: The story of CIA brainwashing experiments in Canada.* Toronto, ON: Lester & Orpen Dennys.

Coons, P. (1994). Confirmation of childhood abuse in child and adolescent cases of multiple personality disorder and dissociative disorder not otherwise specified. *The Journal of Nervous and Mental Disease, 182*(8), 461-464.

Dain, N. (1980). Clifford Beers: An advocate for the insane. Pittsburgh, PA: University of Pittsburgh Press.

Dain, N. (1994). Psychiatry and anti-psychiatry in the United States. In M. Micale & R. Porter, *Discovering the history of psychiatry.* Oxford, UK: Oxford University Press.

Deegan, P. (1990). Spirit breaking: When the helping professions hurt. *The Humanistic Psychologist, 18,* 301-313.

Dewar, G. (1995). Consumer/survivor run alternatives to traditional mental health services: Emphasis on employment for consumer/survivors. *Network.* (Available from the Canadian Mental Health Association, Toronto, ON)

Doerner, K. (1981). *Madmen and the bourgeoisie: A social history of insanity and psychiatry.* New York: Basil Blackwell.

Duerr, M. (1996). *Hearing voices.* Unpublished master's thesis, California Institute of Integral Studies. (Available from the California Institute of Integral Studies, San Francisco, CA)

Dukszta, J. (1987). Research interview conducted at the former Queen Street Mental Health Centre, now part of the Centre for Addiction and Mental Health, Toronto, ON. Unpublished.

Durbin, J., & Sondhu, R. (1992). *Improving mental health supports for diverse ethno/racial communities in Metro Toronto.* (Available from the Metro Toronto District Health Council, Toronto, ON)

Dymond, M., Brown, W., & McNeel, B. (1959). *Proposed revision of mental health programs in Ontario (The Dymond Report).* Toronto, ON: Department of Health.

Estroff, S. (1989). Self, identity and subjective experiences of schizophrenia: In search of a subject. *Schizophrenia Bulletin, 15*(2), 189-196.

Evans, R. (1994). Introduction. In R. Evans, M. Barer, & T. Marmor (Eds.), *Why are some people healthy and others not?* New York: Aldine de Gruyter.

Evans, R., & Stoddart, G. (1994). Producing health, consuming health care. In R. Evans, M. Barer, & T. Marmor (Eds.), *Why are some people healthy and others not?* New York: Aldine de Gruyter.

Evans, R., Barer, M., & Marmor, T. (Eds.). (1994). *Why are some people healthy and others not?* New York: Aldine de Gruyter.

Everett, B. (1994a). Something is happening: The contemporary consumer and psychiatric survivor movement in historical context. *The Journal of Mind and Behaviour, 15*(1-2), 55-70.

Everett, B. (Ed.). (1994b). *You are not alone: A handbook for facilitators of self help and mutual aid groups.* (Available from the Mood Disorders Association, Toronto, ON)

Everett, B., & Shimrat, I. (1993). *Getting mad beats going mad.* Unpublished manuscript. (Available from Homeward, Toronto, ON)

Fight not over yet: Advocacy group calls for boarding home legislation. (1989, November 25). *The Packet and Times.* (Available from the municipal library, Orillia, ON)

Firsten, T. (1991). Violence in the lives of women on psychiatric wards. *Canadian Women's Studies, 11*(4), 45-48.

Foucault, M. (1965). *Madness and civilization: A history of insanity.* New York: Vintage Books.

Foucault, M. (1977). *Power/knowledge: Selected interviews and other writings.* New York: Pantheon Books.

Foucault, M. (1994a). Geneaology and social criticism. In S. Steidman (Ed.), *The Postmodern turn: New perspectives on social theory.* Cambridge, UK: Cambridge University Press.

Foucault, M. (1994b). Two lectures. In M. Kelly (Ed.), *Critique and power: Recasting the Foucault/Habermas debate.* Cambridge, MA: M.I.T. Press.

Freire, P. (1970). *Pedagogy of the oppressed.* New York: Continuum.

Gadacz, R. (1994). *Re-thinking disability: New structures, new relationships.* Edmonton, AB: The University of Alberta Press.

Gamson, W. (1991). Commitment and agency in social movements. *Sociological Forum, 6*(1), 27-50.

Gamson, W. (1995). Hiroshima, the holocaust, and the politics of exclusion. *American Sociological Review, 60*, 1-20.

Gelinas, D. (1983). The persisting negative effects of incest. *Psychiatry, 46*, 312-332.

Gersie, A., & King, N. (1990). *Storymaking in education and therapy*. London, UK: Jessica Kingsley Publishers.

Gil, D. (1996). Preventing violence in a structurally violent society: Mission impossible. *American Journal of Orthopsychiatry, 66*(1), 77-84.

Goff, D., Brotman, D., Kindlon, D., Waites, M., & Amico, E. (1991). Self-reports of childhood abuse in chronically psychotic patients. *Psychiatric Research, 37*(73), 73-80.

Goffman, E. (1961). *Asylums: Essays on the social situation of mental patients and other inmates*. New York: Anchor Books/Doubleday.

Goffman, E. (1963). Notes on the management of a spoiled identity. Englewood Cliffs, NJ: Prentice-Hall.

Goldberg, R. (1991). *Grassroots resistance: Social movements in America*. Belmont, CA: Wadsworth Publishing.

Goodman, L., Dutton, M.A., & Harris, M. (1995). Episodically homeless women with serious mental illness: Prevalence of physical and sexual assault. *American Journal of Orthopsychiatry, 65*(4), 468-478.

Graham, R. (1988). *Building support for people: A plan for mental health in Ontario*. Toronto, ON: Government of Ontario Publication.

Griffin, J. (1989). *In search of sanity: A chronicle of the Canadian Mental Health Association 1918-1988*. (Available from the Ontario Division of the Canadian Mental Health Association, Toronto, ON)

Grob, G. (1991). *From asylum to community: Mental health policy in North America*. Princeton, NJ: Princeton University Press.

Guide to the Substitute Decisions Act, A. (1994). Toronto, ON: Publications Ontario.

Gunderson, M., & Muszynski, L. (1990). *Women and labour market poverty*. Ottawa: The Canadian Advisory Council of the Status of Women.

Handicapped gain new voice. (1992, December 8). *The Packet and Times*. (Available from the municipal library, Orillia, ON)

Hector, R. (1961). *History of Ontario Hospital Queen Street*. Toronto, ON: The Museum of Mental Health Services (Toronto).

Herman, J. (1992). *Trauma and recovery*. New York: Basic Books.

Heseltine, G. (1983). *Towards a blueprint for change: A mental health policy and program perspective*. Toronto, ON: Government of Ontario Publication.

Home's owner jailed for attacks on two handicapped residents. (1988, January 23). *The Toronto Star*. (Available from the Metropolitan Central Reference Library, Toronto, ON)

hooks, b. (1989). *Talking back: Thinking feminist, thinking black*. Toronto, ON: Between the Lines.

Hurst, C. (1990, May). Consumer or survivor? *OPSAnews #1*, pp. 16-17. Toronto, ON: The Ontario Psychiatric Survivors Alliance.

Hutchison, P., Lord, J., & Osbourne-Way, L. (1986). *Participating: Building a framework for support*. Toronto, ON: The Canadian Mental Health Association.

Illich, I. (1975). *Medical nemesis*. London, UK: Ebenezer Bayles & Son.

Immen, W. (1996, July 1). Clinic to open doors for alternative medicine. *The Globe and Mail*, p. 1.

Inquest into the death of Joseph Francis Kendall. (1990). (Copy of the verdict available from the Office of the Chief Coroner, Toronto, ON)

Isaac, R., & Armat, V. (1990). *Madness in the streets: How psychiatry and the law abandoned the mentally ill*. New York: The Free Press.

Janeway, E. (1980). *The power of the weak*. New York: Alfred A. Knopf.

Joffe, R., MacDonald, C., & Kutchner, S. (1989). Life events and mania: A case controlled study. *Psychiatric Research, 30*, 213-216.

Jones, M. (1973). Therapeutic community concepts and the future. In J. Rossi & W. Filstead (Eds.), *The therapeutic community*. New York: Behavioral Publications.

Kalinowsky, L., & Hoch, P. (1961). *Somatic treatments in psychiatry*. New York: Grune & Stratton.

Killian, l. (1964). Social movements. In R. Faris (Ed.), *Handbook of modern sociology* (pp. 426-455). Chicago, IL: Rand NcNally.

Kohler Riessman, C. (1993). *Narrative analyses*. Newbury Park, CA: Sage Publications.

Laing, R.D. (1960). *The divided self*. London, UK: Tavistock Publications.

Leifer, R. (1990). Introduction: The medical model as ideology of the therapeutic state. *The Journal of Mind and Behavior*, *11*(3-4), 247-258.

Lengthy inquest examined plight of home residents. (1991, January 2). *The Packet and Times*. (Available from the municipal library, Orillia, ON)

Leonard, P. (1994). Knowledge/power and postmodernism: Implications for the practice of a critical social work education. *Canadian Social Work Review*, *11*(1), 11-26.

Levin, D. (Ed.). (1971). *Georg Simmel on individuality and social forms*. Chicago, IL: University of Chicago Press.

Levin, M. (1988, Summer). How self help works. *Social Policy*, 39-43.

Lew, M. (1988). *Victims no longer: Men recovering from incest and other sexual child abuse*. New York: Harper & Row.

Life in Orillia's house of horrors. (1988, January 23). *The Toronto Star*. (Available from the Metropolitan Central Reference Library, Toronto, ON)

Lincoln, Y., & Guba, E. (1985). *Naturalist inquiry*. Beverly Hills, CA: Sage Publications.

Lord, J., & Hutchison, P. (1993). The process of empowerment: Implications for theory and practice. *Canadian Journal of Community Mental Health*, *12*(1), 5-22.

Lurie, S. (1984). More for the mind: Have we got less? In *Issues in Canadian human services*. Toronto, ON: OISE Press.

MacNaughton, E. (1992, March). Canadian mental health policy: The emergent picture. *Canada's Mental Health*, pp. 3-10.

Malhotra Bentz, V. (1989). *Becoming mature: Childhood ghosts and spirits in adult life*. New York: Aldine de Gruyter.

Mayer, M. (1991). Social movement research and social movement practice. In D. Rucht (Ed.), *Research on social movements: The state of the art in Western Europe and the U.S.A.* Boulder, CO: Westview Press.

McCracken, G. (1990). *The long interview*. Newbury Park, CA: Sage Publications.

McGuire, M. (1990). The rhetoric of narrative: A hermeneutic, critical theory. In B. Britton & A. Pellegrini (Eds.), *Narrative thought and narrative language*. Hillsdale, NJ: Lawrence Erlbaum Assoc.

McKnight, J. (1994). Community and its counterfeits. CBC radio program *Ideas*. (Transcript available from the CBC, Toronto, ON)

McLean, A. (1990). Contradiction in the social production of clinical knowledge: The case of schizophrenia. *Social Science and Medicine, 30*(9), 969-985.

Melucci, A. (1989) *Nomads of the present*. Philadelphia, PA: Temple University Press.

Melville Whyte, J. (1996). Past the velvet ropes. *Canadian Journal of Community Mental Health, 15*(2), 21-22.

Miller, A. (1981). *The drama of the gifted child*. New York: Basic Books.

Miller, A. (1983). *For your own good: Hidden cruelty in child-rearing and the roots of violence*. New York: Farrar, Straus, Giroux.

Miller, A. (1984). *Thou shalt not be aware: Society's betrayal of the child*. New York: Meridian.

Minkhoff, K. (1987). Beyond deinstitutionalization: A new ideology for the post-institutional era. *Hospital and Community Psychiatry, 38*, 945-950.

Moghadam, V. (1994). Introduction: Women and identity politics in theoretical and comparative perspective. In V. Moghadam (Ed.), *Identity politics and women: Cultural reassertions and feminism in international perspective*. San Francisco, CA: Westview Press.

Monahan, J., & Arnold, J. (1996). Violence by people with mental illness: A consensus statement by advocates and researchers. *Psychiatric Rehabilitation Journal, 19*(4), 67-70.

Muenzenmaier, K., Meyer, I., Struening, E., & Ferker, J. (1993). Childhood abuse and neglect among women outpatients with chronic mental illness. *Hospital and Community Psychiatry, 44*(7), 666-670.

Mullen, P., Martin, J., Anderson, J., Romans, S., & Herbison, G. (1996). The long-term impact of the physical, emotional, and sexual abuse of children: A community study. *Child Abuse and Neglect, 20*(1), 7-21.

Museum of Mental Health Services (Toronto), Inc. (1993). *The city and the asylum*. (Available from the Centre for Addiction and Mental Health, Toronto, ON)

Neidhardt, F., & Rucht, D. (1991). The analysis of social movements: The state of the art and some perspectives for further research. In D. Rucht (Ed.), *Research on social movements: The state of the art in Western Europe and the U.S.A.* Boulder, CO: Westview Press.

Nelson, G., Lord, J., & Ochocka, J. (1996). *Progress Report: Shifting the paradigm in community mental health: A community study of implementation and change: Phase I—Historical policy context.* (Available from the Centre for Research and Education in Human Services, Kitchener, ON)

Newman, D. (1998). *2000 and beyond: Strengthening Ontario's mental health system* [On-line]. Available: http://intra.moh.gov.on.ca/pub/mentalreform.html

Ontario Physicians and Dentists in Public Service (OPDPS). (1994). *Putting people first: Mental health care reform in Ontario: Unresolved issues.* (Available from the OPDPS, Toronto, ON)

OPSAnews #1. (1990, May). Toronto, ON: The Ontario Psychiatric Survivors' Alliance.

OPSAnews #2. (1990, November). Toronto, ON: The Ontario Psychiatric Survivors' Alliance.

OPSAnews #4. (1991, June). Toronto, ON: The Ontario Psychiatric Survivors' Alliance.

OPSAnews #7. (1992, April). Toronto, ON: The Ontario Psychiatric Survivors' Alliance.

OPSEU. (1991). *Care for those who need it: Principles of a comprehensive mental health care system.* (Available from the Ontario Public Service Employees Union, Toronto, ON)

OPSEU. (1994). *Mental health reform in Ontario: Developing our vision.* (Available from the Ontario Public Service Employees Union, Toronto, ON)

Papanek, H. (1994). The ideal woman and the ideal society: Control and autonomy in the construction of identity. In V. Moghadam (Ed.), *Identity politics and women: Cultural reassertions and feminism in international perspective.* San Francisco, CA: Westview Press.

Peat, Marwick & Partners. (1982). *Queen Street Mental Health Centre: An operational and organizational review.*

Penfold, S., & Walker, G. (1983). *Women and the psychiatric paradox.* Montreal: Eden Press.

Pilgrim, D., & Rogers, A. (1993). *A sociology of mental health and illness.* Philadelphia, PA: Open University Press.

Plotke, D. (1995). What's so new about social movements. In S. Lyman (Ed.), *Social movements: Critiques, concepts, case-studies.* Washington Square, NY: New York University Press.

Price, G. (1950). *The development of institutional care and treatment of the mentally ill in Ontario as revealed through the history of the Ontario Hospital, Toronto*. Toronto, ON: The Museum of Mental Health Services (Toronto).

Prilleltensky I., & Gonick, L. (1996). Politics change, oppression remains: On the psychology and politics of oppression. *Political Psychology*, *17*(1), 127-148.

Putting people first: The reform of mental health services in Ontario. (1993). Toronto, ON: Government of Ontario Publication.

Quality of Care Coalition. (1993). *Position paper discussing health services accreditation*. (Available from the Patient Advocate Office, Toronto, ON)

Rachlis, M., & Kushner, C. (1994). *Strong medicine: How to save Canada's health care system*. Toronto, ON: Harper Collins Publishers.

Raibel, C. (1994). "Your daughter and I are not likely to quarrel": Notes on a dispute between Joseph Workman and William Lyon Mackenzie. *Canadian Bulletin of Medical History*, *11*(2), 387-395.

Raymond, V., Lear, D., Bostick, R., Bradford, L., Chamberlin, J., Price, S., & Dumont, J. (1982). *Mental health and violence against women: A feminist ex-inmate analysis*. A brief which resulted from the 10th Annual International Conference on Human Rights and Psychiatric Oppression, Toronto, ON.

Reaume, G. (1994). "Keep your labels off my mind" or "Now I am going to pretend I am crazy but don't be a bit alarmed": Psychiatric history from the patients' perspectives. *Canadian Bulletin of Medical History*, *11*, 397-424.

Report concludes: We can stop group home problems. (1992, October 22). *The Packet and Times*. (Available from the municipal library, Orillia, ON)

Reville, D., & Church, K. (1990). *Doing the right* thing right*. A brief presented to the Toronto hearings of the legislation subcommittee on community mental health services legislation. (Note: As cited in Church, 1993)

Roeher Institute. (1995). *Harm's way: The many faces of violence and abuse against persons with disabilities*. Toronto, ON: The Roeher Institute.

Rosie. (1988). Interview conducted as part of the author's research on the history of the Queen Street Mental Health Centre, Toronto, ON. Unpublished manuscript.

Rothman, D. (1970). *The discovery of the asylum.* Toronto, ON: Little, Brown.

Scheff, T. (1966). *Being mentally ill.* New York: Aldine. (Reprinted in 1984)

Schwartz, D. (1994). Beyond Institutions I. CBC radio program *Ideas.* (Transcript available from CBC Radio, Toronto, ON)

Scull, A. (1979). *Museums of madness: The social organization of insanity in 19th century England.* Markham, ON: Penguin Books.

Shimrat, I. (1989). *Analyzing psychiatry.* (Transcript available from CBC Radio, Toronto, ON)

Shimrat, I. (1997). *Call me crazy: Stories from the mad movement.* Vancouver, BC: Press Gang Publishers.

Showalter, E. (1985). *The female malady: Women, madness and English culture.* New York: Pantheon Books.

Silk, K., Lee, S., Hill, E., & Lohr, N. (1995). Borderline personality disorder symptoms and severity of abuse. *American Journal of Psychiatry, 152*(7), 1059-1064.

Simmons, H. (1990). *Unbalanced: Mental health policy in Ontario, 1930-1989.* Toronto, ON: Wall and Thompson.

Smith, J. (1994). The creation of the world we know: The world economy and the recreation of gendered identities. In V. Moghadam (Ed.), *Identity politics and women: Cultural reassertions and feminism in international perspective.* San Francisco, CA: Westview Press.

Steiner Crane, L., Henson, C., Colliver, J., & MacLean, D. (1988). Prevalence of a history of sexual abuse among female psychiatric patients in a state hospital system. *Hospital and Community Psychiatry, 39*(3), 300-304.

Supeene, S. (1990). *As for the sky, falling: A critical look at psychiatry and suffering.* Toronto, ON: Second Story Press.

Swett, C., Surrey, J., & Cohen, C. (1990). Sexual and physical abuse histories and psychiatric symptoms among male psychiatric outpatients. *American Journal of Psychiatry, 147*(5), 632-636.

System goes too far and not far enough. (1992, December 10). *The Packet and Times.* (Available from the municipal library, Orillia, ON)

Szasz, T. (1974). *The myth of mental illness*. New York: Harper & Row.

Szasz, T. (1989). *Law, liberty and psychiatry*. Syracuse, NY: Syracuse University Press. (Originally published in 1963)

"They erased my memory." How Linda Macdonald rebuilt her life after being brainwashed. (1991, September). *Chatelaine Magazine*, pp. 102, 181

Toffler, A. (1980). *The third wave*. New York: William Morrow.

Toffler, A. (1990). *Powershift*. New York: Bantam Books.

Tories move to repeal. (1995, December 10). *The Toronto Star* (Available from the Metropolitan Central Reference Library, Toronto, ON)

Torrey, E.F. (1995). *Surviving schizophrenia: A manual for families, consumers and providers*. New York: Harper Perennial.

Trainor, J., & Church, K. (1984). *Framework for support of people with severe disabilities*. (Available from the Canadian Mental Health Association, Toronto, ON)

Trainor, J., Church, K., Pape, B., Pomeroy, E., Reville, D., Tefft, B., Lakaski, C., & Renaud, L. (1992, March). Building a framework for support: Developing a sector-based policy model for people with serious mental illness. *Canada's Mental Health*, pp. 25-29.

Tuke, D. (1885). *The insane in the United States and Canada*. New York: Arna Press. (Reprinted in 1973)

Tyhurst, J., Chalke, F., Lawson, F., McNeel, B., Roberts, C., Taylor, G., Weil, R., & Griffin, J. (1963). *More for the mind: A study of psychiatric services in Canada*. Toronto, ON: The Canadian Mental Health Association.

Unzicker, R. (1989). My own: A personal journey through madness and re-emergence. *Psychosocial Rehabilitation Journal, 13*, 71-75.

Van der Kolk, B. (1987). *Psychological trauma*. Washington, DC: American Psychiatric Press.

Van der Kolk, B., & Fisler, R. (1994). Childhood abuse & neglect and loss of self-regulation. *Bulletin of the Menninger Clinic, 58*(2).

W5. (1988). *House of horrors*. (Transcript available from CTV, Toronto, ON)

Wartenberg, T. (1990). *The forms of power: From domination to transformation*. Philadelphia, PA: Temple University Press.

Wigren, J. (1994). Narrative completion in the treatment of trauma. *Psychotherapy, 3*, 415-423.

Wilson, S. (1996). Consumer empowerment in the mental health field. *Canadian Journal of Community Mental Health, 15*(2), 69-85.

Wolfe, N. (1993). *Fire with fire: The new female power and how it will change the 21st century.* Toronto, ON: Random House of Canada.

Zlotnick, C., Ryan, C., Miller, I., & Keitner, G. (1995). Childhood abuse and recovery from major depression. *Child Abuse and Neglect, 19*(12), 1513-1516.

Index